BIRTH DEFECTS

THE ENCYCLOPEDIA OF
H E A L T H

MEDICAL DISORDERS
AND THEIR TREATMENT

Dale C. Garell, M.D. · General Editor

BIRTH DEFECTS

Edward Edelson

Introduction by C. Everett Koop, M.D., Sc.D.
former Surgeon General, U. S. Public Health Service

CHELSEA HOUSE PUBLISHERS

New York · Philadelphia

The goal of the ENCYCLOPEDIA OF HEALTH *is to provide general information in the ever-changing areas of physiology, psychology, and related medical issues. The titles in this series are not intended to take the place of the professional advice of a physician or other health care professional.*

CHELSEA HOUSE PUBLISHERS
EDITOR-IN-CHIEF   Remmel Nunn
MANAGING EDITOR   Karyn Gullen Browne
COPY CHIEF   Mark Rifkin
PICTURE EDITOR   Adrian G. Allen
ART DIRECTOR   Maria Epes
ASSISTANT ART DIRECTOR   Howard Brotman
MANUFACTURING DIRECTOR   Gerald Levine
SYSTEMS MANAGER   Lindsey Ottman
PRODUCTION MANAGER   Joseph Romano
PRODUCTION COORDINATOR   Marie Claire Cebrián

The Encyclopedia of Health
SENIOR EDITOR   Brian Feinberg

Staff for BIRTH DEFECTS
ASSOCIATE EDITOR   LaVonne Carlson-Finnerty
COPY EDITOR   Christopher Duffy
EDITORIAL ASSISTANT   Tamar Levovitz
PICTURE RESEARCHER   Sandy Jones
DESIGNER   Robert Yaffe

First Printing
1   3   5   7   9   8   6   4   2

Library of Congress Cataloging-in-Publication Data

Edelson, Edward.
    Birth defects/by Edward Edelson; introduction by C. Everett Koop.
        p. cm.—(The Encyclopedia of health, medical disorders, and their treatment)
    Includes bibliographical references and index.
    ISBN 0-7910-0058-3
        0-7910-0485-6 (pbk.)
    1. Abnormalities, Human—Juvenile literature. 2. Genetic disorders—Juvenile literature. I. Title. II. Series.
RG626.E34 1992   91-27448
616'.042—dc20   CIP

CONTENTS

THE ENCYCLOPEDIA OF H E A L T H

PREVENTION AND EDUCATION: THE KEYS TO GOOD HEALTH

C. Everett Koop, M.D., Sc.D.
former Surgeon General,
U.S. Public Health Service

The issue of health education has received particular attention in recent years because of the presence of AIDS in the news. But our response to this particular tragedy points up a number of broader issues that doctors, public health officials, educators, and the public face. In particular, it points up the necessity for sound health education for citizens of all ages.

Over the past 25 years this country has been able to bring about dramatic declines in the death rates for heart disease, stroke, accidents, and for people under the age of 45, cancer. Today, Americans generally eat better and take better care of themselves than ever before. Thus, with the help of modern science and technology, they have a better chance of surviving serious—even catastrophic—illnesses. That's the good news.

But, like every phonograph record, there's a flip side, and one with special significance for young adults. According to a report issued in 1979 by Dr. Julius Richmond, my predecessor as Surgeon General, Americans aged 15 to 24 had a higher death rate in 1979 than they did 20 years earlier. The causes: violent death and injury, alcohol and drug abuse, unwanted pregnancies, and sexually transmitted diseases. Adolescents are particularly vulnerable because they are beginning to explore their own sexuality and perhaps to experiment with drugs. The need for educating young people is critical, and the price of neglect is high.

Yet even for the population as a whole, our health is still far from what it could be. Why? A 1974 Canadian government report attributed all death and disease to four broad elements: inadequacies in the health care system, behavioral factors or unhealthy life-styles, environmental hazards, and human biological factors.

To be sure, there are diseases that are still beyond the control of even our advanced medical knowledge and techniques. And despite yearnings that are as old as the human race itself, there is no "fountain of youth" to ward off aging and death. Still, there is a solution to many of the problems that undermine sound health. In a word, that solution is prevention. Prevention, which includes health promotion and education, saves lives, improves the quality of life, and in the long run, saves money.

In the United States, organized public health activities and preventive medicine have a long history. Important milestones in this country or foreign breakthroughs adopted in the United States include the improvement of sanitary procedures and the development of pasteurized milk in the late 19th century and the introduction in the mid-20th century of effective vaccines against polio, measles, German measles, mumps, and other once-rampant diseases. Internationally, organized public health efforts began on a wide-scale basis with the International Sanitary Conference of 1851, to which 12 nations sent representatives. The World Health Organization, founded in 1948, continues these efforts under the aegis of the United Nations, with particular emphasis on combating communicable diseases and the training of health care workers.

Despite these accomplishments, much remains to be done in the field of prevention. For too long, we have had a medical care system that is science- and technology-based, focused, essentially, on illness and mortality. It is now patently obvious that both the social and the economic costs of such a system are becoming insupportable.

Implementing prevention—and its corollaries, health education and promotion—is the job of several groups of people.

First, the medical and scientific professions need to continue basic scientific research, and here we are making considerable progress. But increased concern with prevention will also have a decided impact on how primary care doctors practice medicine. With a shift to health-based rather than morbidity-based medicine, the role of the "new physician" will include a healthy dose of patient education.

Second, practitioners of the social and behavioral sciences— psychologists, economists, city planners—along with lawyers, business leaders, and government officials—must solve the practical and ethical dilemmas confronting us: poverty, crime, civil rights, literacy, education, employment, housing, sanitation, environmental protection, health care delivery systems, and so forth. All of these issues affect public health.

Third is the public at large. We'll consider that very important group in a moment.

Fourth, and the linchpin in this effort, is the public health profession—doctors, epidemiologists, teachers—who must harness the professional expertise of the first two groups and the common sense and cooperation of the third, the public. They must define the problems statistically and qualitatively and then help us set priorities for finding the solutions.

To a very large extent, improving those statistics is the responsibility of every individual. So let's consider more specifically what the role of the individual should be and why health education is so important to that role. First, and most obvious, individuals can protect themselves from illness and injury and thus minimize their need for professional medical care. They can eat nutritious food; get adequate exercise; avoid tobacco, alcohol, and drugs; and take prudent steps to avoid accidents. The proverbial "apple a day keeps the doctor away" is not so far from the truth, after all.

Second, individuals should actively participate in their own medical care. They should schedule regular medical and dental checkups. Should they develop an illness or injury, they should know when to treat themselves and when to seek professional help. To gain the maximum benefit from any medical treatment that they do require, individuals must become partners in that treatment. For instance, they should understand the effects and side effects of medications. I counsel young physicians that there is no such thing as too much information when talking with patients. But the corollary is the patient must know enough about the nuts and bolts of the healing process to understand what the doctor is telling him or her. That is at least partially the patient's responsibility.

Education is equally necessary for us to understand the ethical and public policy issues in health care today. Sometimes individuals will encounter these issues in making decisions about their own treatment or that of family members. Other citizens may encounter them as jurors in medical malpractice cases. But we all become involved, indirectly, when we elect our public officials, from school board members to the president. Should surrogate parenting be legal? To what extent is drug testing desirable, legal, or necessary? Should there be public funding for family planning, hospitals, various types of medical research, and other medical care for the indigent? How should we allocate scant technological resources, such as kidney dialysis and organ transplants? What is the proper role of government in protecting the rights of patients?

What are the broad goals of public health in the United States today? In 1980, the Public Health Service issued a report aptly entitled *Promoting Health—Preventing Disease: Objectives for the Nation*. This report expressed its goals in terms of mortality and in terms of intermediate goals in education and health improvement. It identified 15 major concerns: controlling high blood pressure; improving family planning; improving pregnancy care and infant health; increasing the rate of immunization; controlling sexually transmitted diseases; controlling the presence of toxic agents and radiation in the environment; improving occupational safety and health; preventing accidents; promoting water fluoridation and dental health; controlling infectious diseases; decreasing smoking; decreasing alcohol and drug abuse; improving nutrition; promoting physical fitness and exercise; and controlling stress and violent behavior.

For healthy adolescents and young adults (ages 15 to 24), the specific goal was a 20% reduction in deaths, with a special focus on motor vehicle injuries and alcohol and drug abuse. For adults (ages 25 to 64), the aim was 25% fewer deaths, with a concentration on heart attacks, strokes, and cancers.

Smoking is perhaps the best example of how individual behavior can have a direct impact on health. Today, cigarette smoking is recognized as the single most important preventable cause of death in our society. It is responsible for more cancers and more cancer deaths than any other known agent; is a prime risk factor for heart and blood vessel disease, chronic bronchitis, and emphysema; and is a frequent cause of complications in pregnancies and of babies born prematurely, underweight, or with potentially fatal respiratory and cardiovascular problems.

Since the release of the Surgeon General's first report on smoking in 1964, the proportion of adult smokers has declined substantially, from 43% in 1965 to 30.5% in 1985. Since 1965, 37 million people have quit smoking. Although there is still much work to be done if we are to become a "smoke-free society," it is heartening to note that public health and public education efforts—such as warnings on cigarette packages and bans on broadcast advertising—have already had significant effects.

In 1835, Alexis de Tocqueville, a French visitor to America, wrote, "In America the passion for physical well-being is general." Today, as then, health and fitness are front-page items. But with the greater scientific and technological resources now available to us, we are in a far stronger position to make good health care available to everyone. And with the greater technological threats to us as we approach the 21st century, the need to do so is more urgent than ever before. Comprehensive information about basic biology, preventive medicine, medical and surgical treatments, and related ethical and public policy issues can help you arm yourself with the knowledge you need to be healthy throughout your life.

FOREWORD

Dale C. Garell, M.D.

Advances in our understanding of health and disease during the 20th century have been truly remarkable. Indeed, it could be argued that modern health care is one of the greatest accomplishments in all of human history. In the early 20th century, improvements in sanitation, water treatment, and sewage disposal reduced death rates and increased longevity. Previously untreatable illnesses can now be managed with antibiotics, immunizations, and modern surgical techniques. Discoveries in the fields of immunology, genetic diagnosis, and organ transplantation are revolutionizing the prevention and treatment of disease. Modern medicine is even making inroads against cancer and heart disease, two of the leading causes of death in the United States.

Although there is much to be proud of, medicine continues to face enormous challenges. Science has vanquished diseases such as smallpox and polio, but new killers, most notably AIDS, confront us. Moreover, we now victimize ourselves with what some have called "diseases of choice," or those brought on by drug and alcohol abuse, bad eating habits, and mismanagement of the stresses and strains of contemporary life. The very technology that is doing so much to prolong life has brought with it previously unimaginable ethical dilemmas related to issues of death and dying. The rising cost of health care is a matter of central concern to us all. And violence in the form of automobile accidents, homicide, and suicide remains the major killer of young adults.

In the past, most people were content to leave health care and medical treatment in the hands of professionals. But since the 1960s, the consumer of medical care—that is, the patient—has assumed an increasingly central role in the management of his or her own health. There has also been a new emphasis placed on prevention: People are recognizing that their own actions can help prevent many of the conditions that have caused death and disease in the past. This accounts for the growing commitment to good nutrition and regular exercise, for the increasing number of people who are choosing not to smoke, and for a new moderation in people's drinking habits.

People want to know more about themselves and their own health. They are curious about their body: its anatomy, physiology, and biochemistry. They want to keep up with rapidly evolving medical technologies and procedures. They are willing to educate themselves about common disorders and diseases so that they can be full partners in their own health care.

THE ENCYCLOPEDIA OF HEALTH is designed to provide the basic knowledge that readers will need if they are to take significant responsibility for their own health. It is also meant to serve as a frame of reference for further study and exploration. The encyclopedia is divided into five subsections: The Healthy Body; The Life Cycle; Medical Disorders & Their Treatment; Psychological Disorders & Their Treatment; and Medical Issues. For each topic covered by the encyclopedia, we present the essential facts about the relevant biology; the symptoms, diagnosis, and treatment of common diseases and disorders; and ways in which you can prevent or reduce the severity of health problems when that is possible. The encyclopedia also projects what may lie ahead in the way of future treatment or prevention strategies.

The broad range of topics and issues covered in the encyclopedia reflects that human health encompasses physical, psychological, social, environmental, and spiritual well-being. Just as the mind and the body are inextricably linked, so, too, is the individual an integral part of the wider world that comprises his or her family, society, and environment. To discuss health in its broadest aspect it is necessary to explore the many ways in which it is connected to such fields as law, social science, public policy, economics, and even religion. And so, the encyclopedia is meant to be a bridge between science, medical technology, the world at large, and you. I hope that it will inspire you to pursue in greater depth particular areas of interest and that you will take advantage of the suggestions for further reading and the lists of resources and organizations that can provide additional information.

CHAPTER 1

AN OVERVIEW OF BIRTH DEFECTS

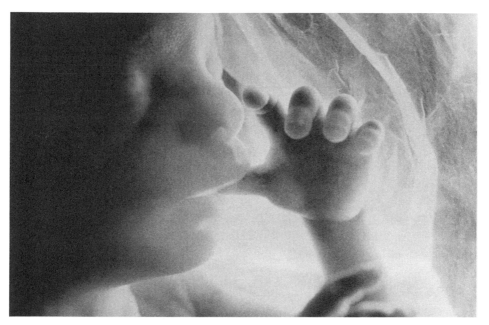

Creation of human life is a complex process. Usually, fetal development progresses smoothly, but major errors can occur. It is believed that 2% to 3% of all babies born in the United States each year suffer from a prominent birth defect.

Assembling a human being from a single fertilized egg is a formidable task. Nature does not always do the job perfectly, and the result is that 2% to 3% of all babies born in the United States have a major malformation, according to the March of Dimes Birth Defects Foundation. Some defects, moreover, became apparent later in childhood, as they emerge during the process of mental and physical development. However, although statistics can demonstrate the importance of science's battle against birth defects, they should not frighten those considering parenthood. Indeed, the vast majority of infants delivered each year are perfectly healthy. Altogether, more than 4 million babies were born in the United States in 1989, according to the federal Centers for Disease Control (CDC).

Defining a birth defect is not always a simple matter. Some defects are obvious, but others, including inherited risks for disease, are not always classified as birth defects. Whether learning disabilities should be categorized as birth defects is particularly problematic because it has been difficult to pinpoint their causes. For example, *dyslexia*, a learning disorder that affects the ability to read, appears to have a strong genetic component. In the early years of the 20th century, studies in Sweden found that most dyslexic children came from families in which other members had reading problems. The condition also has a strong sexual bias: For every girl with dyslexia, there are at least four boys with the condition. Although it is not known for certain why, one theory suggests that the disorder may result from the fetus's reaction to the male hormone testosterone.

For the purpose of this book, the definition of birth defect will include a broad range of problems—physical and genetic abnormalities and defects in the body's chemistry—present at birth.

A WIDESPREAD PROBLEM

Because medical science has conquered most of the common diseases of childhood, birth defects have become an increasing focus in newborn and pediatric medicine and have emerged as the leading cause of

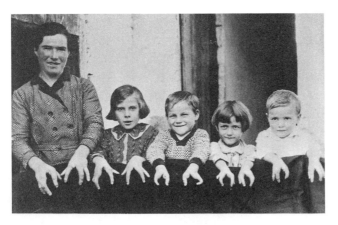

Genetic defects, such as this one found in a mother and her children, are the result of abnormal genes passed from parent to offspring.

major childhood hospitalizations and deaths in the United States and other developed countries.

According to a report from the CDC, birth defects were an underlying cause of death for more than 9,000 of the almost 39,000 babies who died before their first birthday in the United States in 1986. Birth defects thus were responsible for more than 23% of those deaths, more than any other cause.

The CDC also estimates that abnormalities of the heart and blood vessels are linked to 38% of infant deaths, making them the leading cause of infant mortality. Abnormalities of the central nervous system (brain and spinal cord) are second, occurring in almost 15% of infant deaths, and respiratory system defects, found in almost 11% of cases, are the third leading cause of mortality.

EXAMPLES

Heart defects are common, occurring in 1 of every 120 births, according to the March of Dimes. The organ begins to form about the third week of pregnancy from a single tube that contorts and divides, eventually creating a multichambered pump. Because the process is so complex, it is not surprising that mistakes occur. In the case of a *ventricular septal defect*, for example, there is a hole between the two lower pumping chambers of the heart. In other cases, the artery that connects the heart and the lungs is abnormally narrow, a problem known as *pulmonary stenosis*. Another condition, called *tetralogy of Fallot*, consists of a number of heart defects in the same child. An infant suffering from this is called a *blue baby* because a circulation problem in the heart causes some of the infant's blood to bypass the lungs where it would pick up needed oxygen for the rest of the body. As a result, the infant takes on a bluish pallor. (Many other heart problems also result in blue babies.) Surgery often is needed to save the child or to allow him or her to develop normally. In fact, many open-heart surgery techniques now used for adults with heart disease were pioneered for babies with congenital (present at birth) heart defects.

In the digestive tract, defects range from *esophageal atresia* (incomplete formation of the esophagus, the tube that carries food from

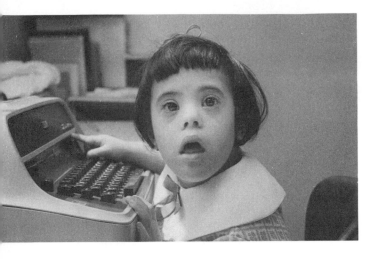

Down's syndrome is usually caused by the presence of an extra chromosome 21 in a developing fetus. It results in mental retardation and physical defects.

the throat to the stomach) to blockages or malformations of different portions of the small or large intestine. Many of these intestinal defects are fatal unless surgery is performed to correct them. The causes of most of them are unknown.

When several birth defects often occur together to form a distinct pattern, they are collectively called a *syndrome*. For example, children with *Down's syndrome*, which leads to mental retardation, often have congenital heart defects as well as other physical abnormalities. Hundreds of syndromes have been identified.

TYPES OF BIRTH DEFECTS

In recent decades, biomedical research has solved some of the mysteries behind birth defects, information that has helped produce new methods for preventing and treating abnormalities. Yet much remains to be learned. The causes of most birth defects are still poorly understood.

Even so, current knowledge allows many defects to be classified by their cause:

- *Hereditary birth defects* result from harmful *genes* (which contain the genetic code for life) passed from parent to child.

- *Chromosomal birth defects* occur when a fetus has too many or too few chromosomes (structures in a cell that hold genes) or possesses a chromosome with an abnormal structure.

- *Environmental birth defects*, also known as *acquired birth defects*, are caused by factors that act on the fetus in the womb, such as radiation or toxic chemicals to which the mother may be exposed.
- *Multifactorial birth defects*, a particularly complex and baffling group of abnormalities, occur when genes interact with environmental factors to produce defects.

An impressive amount of progress has been made in the field of hereditary birth defects, especially those caused by just one gene. More than 4,000 such single-gene defects have been identified, and the number continues to grow.

Research also has led to a better understanding of chromosomal defects, the most prominent of these being Down's syndrome. This condition is usually caused by the presence of an extra chromosome and, as mentioned, leads to a distinct pattern of major and minor defects, including mental retardation. People with extra, missing, or abnormal chromosomes are all at risk for birth defects.

Contributing Factors

About 10% of birth defects are caused by environmental and life-style factors—infections, chemicals, diseases of the mother, and other outside influences that affect the fetus as it develops in the womb. Alcohol consumption and drug use are the leading causes of such defects. Sometimes the effect is direct and unmistakable, as in the case of the severe defects caused by the drug *thalidomide*, which interferes with normal development of the arms and legs of the fetus when taken during pregnancy, and can cause ear and cardiac defects as well.

Continuing Questions

In a large percentage of cases, however, the exact cause of birth defects remains unknown. Although there is a great deal of evidence that many defects are caused by an interaction between genetic and environmental factors, in the majority of cases—perhaps 60%—it is impossible to identify the precise cause. One of the great challenges for science is to reduce the uncertainty regarding the cause of many birth defects.

Such is the case with a group of conditions called *neural tube defects*, in which the spinal cord and brain do not develop normally. One example is *anencephaly*, in which most or all of the brain is missing; it usually results in *stillbirth* (in which the infant is dead at birth) or causes death within a short time. Another such defect is *spina bifida*, in which the bone surrounding the spinal cord does not close completely; it can cause a variety of problems, including the inability to control the bowels or bladder, trouble moving, and paralysis. The incidence of neural tube defects in the United States is 1 out of every 1,000 births, according to the CDC. In Northern Ireland, however, such defects occur in 3 out of every 1,000 births. A high incidence has also been found in India and Alexandria, Egypt. It is not known whether geographic location, genetic characteristics, or social factors, such as

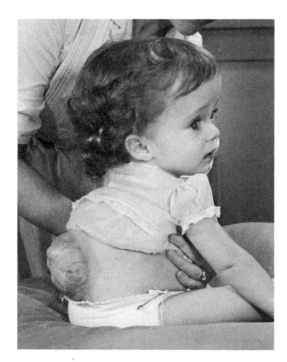

Spina bifida, a defect in which the bone surrounding the spinal cord does not close completely, can result in a number of medical problems, including paralysis. Like many other birth defects, the precise cause of this condition remains unclear.

poverty and a poor diet, are responsible for these occurrences. (A recent study, however, indicates that folic acid, administered under a doctor's supervision to women prior to and in the early part of pregnancy, may help prevent spina bifida.)

PREDICTING BIRTH DEFECTS

A better understanding of the genetic and environmental factors behind birth defects will help researchers predict the chance of such problems when a couple sets out to have a child. It is already clear that some defects run in families. This does not mean that every member of the family is affected but that the chance of a defect occurring is higher than average. In an analysis of families plagued by birth defects, Dr. Cedric Carter of the Hospital for Sick Children in London looked at a number of problems such as *cleft palate* (in which bones in the palate do not fuse during the development of the fetus, leaving a cleft, or opening, in the roof of the mouth; this can cause speech and swallowing difficulties unless it is corrected) and neural tube and congenital heart defects. His research suggested that if one parent is affected by the condition, the risk of having a child with that defect is 3% to 5%. If neither parent is affected but they have one child with the defect, the risk for later births may run from 2% to 5%. In a family with three affected children, the risk of recurrence in later births could rise to 25%.

Many such studies also show that there is a relationship between gender—either of the child or the parents—and the risk of a specific defect. Only boys, for example, can be afflicted by *Duchenne muscular dystrophy*, which causes a progessive wasting away of the muscles.

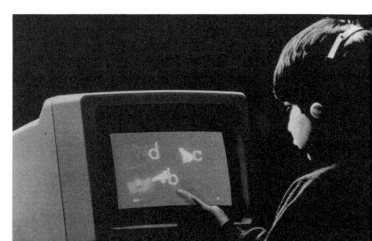

The learning disorder dyslexia occurs primarily in males; one theory suggests that this may be related to the fetus's reaction to the male hormone testosterone.

Hemophilia (a disease in which the blood will not clot properly, so that even a minor injury can cause severe bleeding) also occurs almost exclusively in males. In other cases, the role gender plays is less obvious. For example, a woman born with the intestinal malformation called *pyloric stenosis* (in which the opening between the stomach and the small intestine is abnormally narrow or obstructed) has a 7% risk of bearing a daughter with that defect; the risk of bearing a son with the condition is greater than 16%. A father born with pyloric stenosis has a 5% chance of having an affected son and a 2.5% chance of having a daughter with that condition.

INHERITING AN INCREASED RISK

Not all inherited problems are easily classified as birth defects, however. Some families pass on genes that have no immediate effect on their offspring but do give that child an increased risk of developing a disease later in life. Type II diabetes, a form of the disease that generally occurs in adulthood, is one example. A person's chances of developing it are considered higher if other members of the family have it as well. Heart disease, which often runs in families and generally does not strike until the middle years of life, is another example. In addition, a few kinds of cancer have a strong genetic component; one of these is *retinoblastoma*, which affects the eyes. Another example is breast cancer. A woman with one or more close relatives (a mother or sister, for example) who have had breast cancer is at higher risk of getting the disease herself. Depending upon her age and the number of close relatives who have had the disease, the woman's risk may be two to five times higher than normal.

Even so, just because an individual is more likely than most people to get a specific illness does not mean that this will happen. Various nongenetic factors, including diet and other habits, can play a part as well. For example, although heredity is considered to be one factor behind Type II diabetes, doctors have evidence that obesity also contributes to this condition. In the case of heart disease, heredity must again share the blame with other culprits, including foods high in fat and cholesterol.

CHAPTER 2

GENETIC DEFECTS

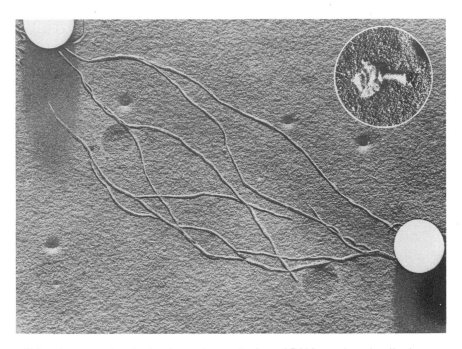

This microscopic photo shows long chains of DNA, molecules that contain the genetic code of life. The virus particle from which this DNA was extracted is also pictured.

Human beings have close to 100,000 genes per cell, which carry all the information needed for the body to develop and function. Each human has two sets of genes, one from the mother and one from the father. Because genetic factors play a major role in the development of birth defects, it is essential to understand the basics of genetics in any discussion of defects.

GENES AND CHROMOSOMES

A gene is a section of a very large molecule called DNA, or *deoxyribonucleic acid*. DNA is made up of molecular units called *nucleotides*, each of which contains a sugar molecule (in this case deoxyribose sugar), a *phosphate group* (phosphorous with oxygen atoms attached), and one of four *bases*: *adenine*, *cytosine*, *guanine*, or *thymine*, abbreviated A, C, G, and T. The bases are linked together into an enormously long chain.

The body's DNA is stored inside a protective wrapping of protein. This DNA-protein structure is the *chromosome*, and a human cell contains 46 (23 pairs) of them. Chromosomes were first discovered in the late 19th century when scientists peering through their microscopes noted that if they added a dye when a cell divided, small, threadlike bodies absorbed the dye and became visible. The scientists called these objects chromosomes, from the Greek words for "colored bodies." There are actually two strands of nucleotides per DNA molecule, linked together and twisted into a shape something like a spiral staircase. This shape is called a *double helix*. The rungs of the staircase are formed by pairs of bases. Adenine always pairs with thymine and guanine always pairs with cytosine. The sizes of the bases are such that an AT pair is just as long as a CG pair, so the width of the DNA double helix is uniform.

Added together, all the DNA in a human cell has three billion base pairs. Most of the cells of the body contain the full complement of DNA (among the few exceptions are red blood cells), and the code of life is contained in the sequence of base pairs. The genetic code can be compared to Morse code, in which specific sequences of dots and dashes are translated into letters. The genetic codes consist of three-base units that, through a complicated process carried out inside the cell, are translated into molecules called *amino acids*. For example, the sequence CGA codes for an amino acid called arginine, the sequence ACC codes for an amino acid called threonine, and the sequence CCC codes for the amino acid proline. Amino acids combine to form proteins, which carry out the essential functions of life. A gene, specifically, is a portion of a DNA molecule that contains the code for an entire protein.

The Structure of DNA

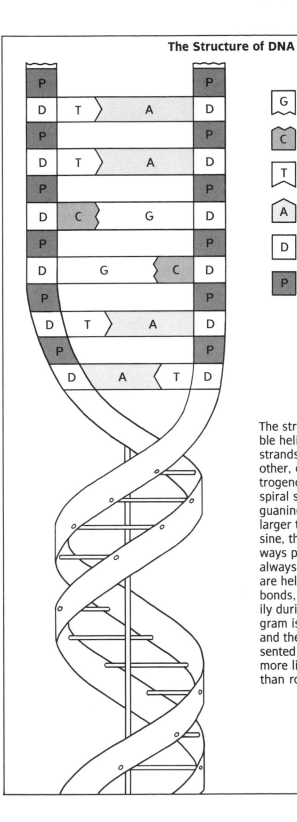

G	guanine
C	cytosine
T	thymine
A	adenine
D	deoxyribose
P	phosphate

The structure of DNA is a double helix: two phosphate-sugar strands wrapped around each other, connected by paired nitrogenous bases, much like a spiral staircase. Adenine and guanine, the purines, are larger than thymine and cytosine, the pyrimidines. A always pairs with T, and G always pairs with C. The bases are held together by hydrogen bonds, which come apart easily during replication. This diagram is not drawn to scale, and the base pairs, represented by rods, are actually more like flat "steps" than rods.

Every human being starts out as a single cell with, as mentioned, a set of genes from each parent. That cell divides, and its *daughter cells* divide again and again; the DNA reproduces itself at each division. With this growth of cells comes specialization into nerve cells, skin cells, and all the other cells of the body. Every cell division means reproduction of the full complement of genes; specialization means that some genes are turned off in some cells so those cells can carry out their specific functions in the body. The genes that are active in a nerve cell are not the same as the genes that are active in a muscle cell.

GENETIC ERRORS

There are many ways in which genes can go wrong in this endless process of reproduction. Indeed, human beings and all other living creatures on this planet would not be here were it not for these genetic errors. Evolution depends on changes, or *mutations*, in genetic material, since some provide useful new characteristics that allow species to arise.

Many things can cause errors in gene reproduction. One example is a *point mutation*, in which one base in a gene is replaced with another, causing a change in the protein code. Perhaps the most famous point mutation (because it was among the first to be discovered and affects

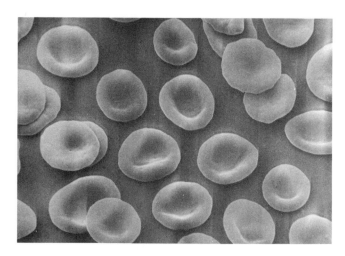

Blood cells from a sickle-cell anemia victim. The condition results when a small change in a gene causes the amino acid valine to replace glutamic acid in the protein hemoglobin. The mutated gene occurs in 1 out of 12 of African Americans.

so many people) is the one that causes the amino acid called *valine* to replace one called *glutamic acid* in the chain of 146 amino acids that form the oxygen-carrying protein called *hemoglobin*, found in red blood cells. That seemingly small change alters the structure of hemoglobin in a way that leads to the blood disease *sickle-cell anemia*, which can prove fatal. This mutated gene occurs in about 1 out of 12 Americans of African origin; about 1 out of every 500 have the disease, according to a 1973 report in the *New England Journal of Medicine*.

TYPES OF GENETIC BIRTH DEFECTS

Genetic diseases and defects usually are defined by the way in which they are inherited. One class of disease or defect is caused by a single mutated gene that can be inherited from either parent. This form of inheritance is called *dominant* because the gene can cancel out the effects of the nonmutated gene inherited from the other parent. Another form of inheritance is called *recessive* because the disease or defect

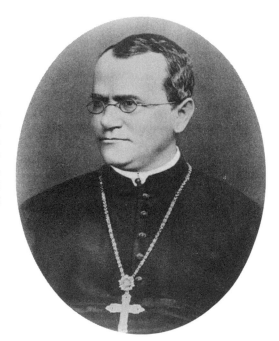

By crossbreeding different strains of pea plants and studying the various traits they passed on, Austrian monk Gregor Mendel (1822–84) discovered the laws of genetics.

25

occurs only if the individual inherits the same two mutated genes, one from each parent. In this case, an individual who inherits only one altered gene does not have the condition because the gene from the other parent is sufficient for normal functioning.

A third form, *sex-linked* inheritance, has to do with two specific chromosomes. As previously noted, human cells have 23 pairs of chromosomes. However, only one pair determines the sex of a developing fetus. A female has two *X chromosomes*, so called because of their shape. A male has an X chromosome and a *Y chromosome*. The Y chromosome is much smaller than the X and contains few genes. Thus, it is just about certain that a mutated gene on the X chromosome will not have a matching gene on the Y chromosome to correct for the defect. A number of genetic conditions therefore occur only or primarily in males, including Duchenne muscular dystrophy, hemophilia and color blindness, the result of a recessive gene that causes the development of defective color receptors in the eye.

Dominant Gene Defects

About 2,000 disorders are caused by dominant genes. One of the best-known dominant disorders is *Huntington's chorea*, which causes a progressive, fatal degeneration of the nervous system that usually begins in the middle years of life. Another is *achondroplastic dwarfism*, which is characterized by an underlying skeletal defect that results in stature under five feet tall. Still another is *Marfan syndrome*. Patients with this condition are tall and lean; some have defects of the eyes, bones, and blood vessels due to abnormalities in the body's connective tissue. There is some evidence, though far from conclusive, that Abraham Lincoln suffered from the condition.

One of the most intriguing dominant disorders is called *familial hypercholesterolemia*, which causes unusually high blood cholesterol levels. One out of every 500 Americans carries the gene for this condition, which reduces the ability of cells to dispose of cholesterol in the blood. The result is an unusually quick buildup of fatty deposits that clog the coronary arteries, causing heart attacks. The study of individuals with familial hypercholesterolemia has led to important

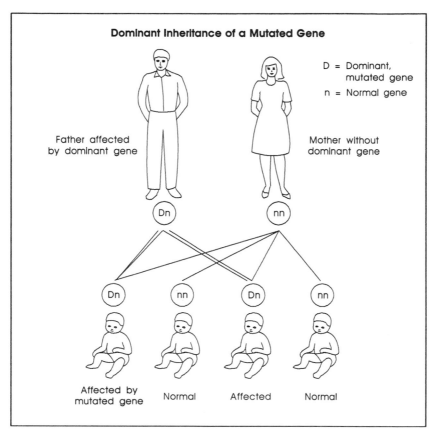

D = Dominant, mutated gene

n = Normal gene

Father affected by dominant gene

Mother without dominant gene

Dn

nn

Dn

nn

Dn

nn

Affected by mutated gene

Normal

Affected

Normal

Dominant inheritance occurs when a single gene passed down from a child's mother or father causes a trait to appear.

advances in knowledge of the way that high blood cholesterol levels cause heart disease. There are several other dominant gene defects that are also linked to blood cholesterol and fat levels. Together, these gene-related problems affect 1 out of every 100 Americans and thus are important factors in heart disease, the leading cause of death in the United States.

Recessive Gene Defects

Recessive inheritance is not as simple to explain as dominant traits are, but arithmetic can help to illustrate the process. Every human is believed to carry perhaps 8 to 12 harmful recessive genes. Suppose two people who carry the same harmful recessive gene have a child. Each egg from the mother and sperm from the father carries only one set of genes instead of the two sets that other cells have (this will be discussed further in Chapter 3). Half the eggs and half the sperm carry the nonharmful gene; the other half carry the mutated gene. It is a matter of pure chance whether the egg and the sperm that unite to make an embryo carry the nonmutated gene or the mutated recessive gene. Therefore, an embryo has one chance in four of inheriting two non-harmful genes. It has two chances in four of inheriting one nonmutated and one altered gene and one chance in four of inheriting two mutated genes. Thus, when both parents carry one mutated recessive gene, there is a 25% risk each time they have a child that the baby will have that genetic defect.

For a recessive trait to appear, a gene for that condition must be in-herited from both parents.

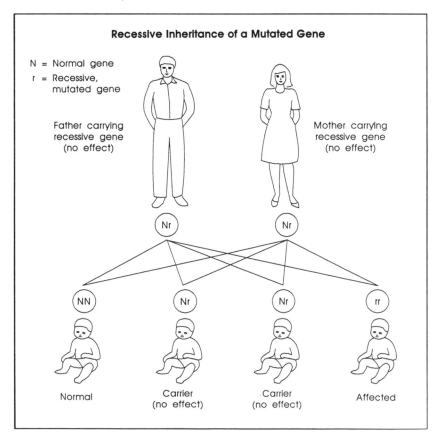

Recessive Inheritance of a Mutated Gene

N = Normal gene
r = Recessive, mutated gene

Father carrying recessive gene (no effect)

Mother carrying recessive gene (no effect)

Nr   Nr

NN   Nr   Nr   rr

Normal   Carrier   Carrier   Affected
            (no effect) (no effect)

The frequency of certain mutated recessive genes is especially high in particular populations. In some cases, the reason is known. A single recessive gene for sickle-cell anemia protects against a virulent form of malaria found in certain parts of Africa. The protective function of that gene for the entire population outweighed the damage done to those who inherited two sickle-cell anemia genes. The same is true of a closely related set of conditions called *thalassemias*, found in people from Mediterranean regions where malaria is also a threat.

Other ailments caused by recessive genes include *Tay-Sachs disease*, a condition that affects the brain and can cause paralysis, blindness, and mental retardation. The disorder can ultimately result in death two to five years after birth. It is caused by a lack of the enzyme *hexosamidase A*, which helps break down fat. The Tay-Sachs gene is carried by 4% of Jews of eastern European origin. The most common recessive condition in American whites is *cystic fibrosis*, characterized by an unusually thick, sticky mucus that causes chronic infections and problems absorbing food. One out of every 25 white Americans carries the gene for cystic fibrosis. Simple arithmetic can predict the incidence of the disease. There is 1 chance in 625 (25 times 25) that both parents in the general white population will be carriers of the cystic fibrosis gene. Each child of such a couple will have one chance in four of inheriting both recessive genes. The incidence of cystic fibrosis is thus 1 in 4 times 625, or 1 in every 2,500 births.

It is also important to note that although the incidence of recessive genes is higher in some populations and ethnic groups, just about anyone can have a condition caused by a harmful recessive gene. Having an affected child is not a sign of inferiority but simply a matter of how the genetic dice are rolled. Some 1,400 recessive genetic disorders have been identified. Most affect only a few people; some have been found only in a single family.

Another point to keep in mind is that, although this text concentrates on birth defects and therefore deals with deleterious genes, dominant and recessive inheritance often involve genes that are not harmful at all, or actually provide a benefit. For example, a person's freckles, dimples, eye color, hair color, and blood type are all determined by dominant or recessive genes.

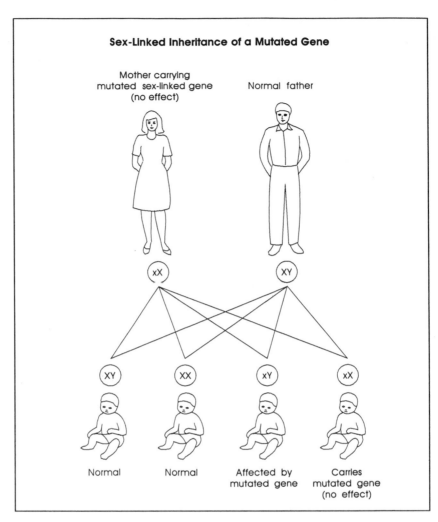

Sex-Linked Inheritance of a Mutated Gene

Mother carrying
mutated sex-linked gene
(no effect)

Normal father

xX

XY

XY

XX

xY

xX

Normal

Normal

Affected by
mutated gene

Carries
mutated gene
(no effect)

A mutated gene carried on the X chromosome often results in sex-linked inheritance, a problem occurring most often in males. Because females inherit two X chromosomes, a mutated gene on one of them is usually canceled out by a nonmutated gene on the other.

Sex-Linked Birth Defects

Many disorders are caused by mutated genes on the X chromosome. A girl who inherits such a gene usually has a matching, but nonmutated, gene on her other X and so is unaffected by the mutation, but a boy's small Y chromosome will probably not have a counteracting gene. The most common X-linked disorder is color blindness. One form, *red-green blindness*, in which an individual has trouble recognizing red and green affects 1 in 12 white males.

However, there are rare occasions when a female can develop an X-linked disorder—when she is the child of a male with the condition and a female who carries the gene for the disorder, for example. More commonly, though, a female carries the mutated gene on just one chromosome and shows a limited effect from it because the nonmutated gene on the other X chromosome does not make up fully for the mutated one. For example, a woman who carries the Duchenne muscular dystrophy gene may have muscle weakness and a woman who carries the hemophilia gene may have slower blood clotting. These symptoms make themselves felt because one of the two X chromosomes in every cell, of a female's body is inactivated early in life. If enough X chromosomes carrying the nonmutated gene are inactivated, signs of the disease become evident.

It has also been found that some people who inherit mutated dominant genes do not develop all the symptoms of a condition. Geneticists call this phenomenon *incomplete penetrance*. Some people with the dominant condition *neurofibromatosis* (mistakenly known as Elephant Man disease, although John Merrick, the 19th-century Briton about whom a play and movie were written, actually had a related condition called Proteus disease) have curvature of the spine and many tumors. Others have only a few skin lesions. Scientists as yet cannot explain incomplete penetrance.

Multifactorial Birth Defects

Another large category of genetically related defects are those that are caused not by a single gene but by a number of genes interacting with environmental factors. In this case, the faulty genes inherited by the fetus are not, by themselves, necessarily enough to cause a defect. They only increase the chance that the defect will occur. There must also be some outside influence on the fetus—perhaps if the mother is taking certain drugs or is not getting proper nutrition while she is pregnant—before the scale is ultimately tipped toward a birth defect.

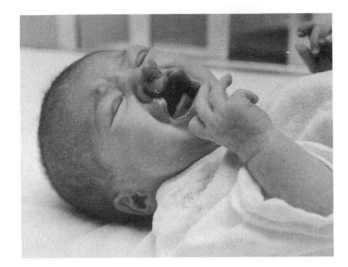

Cleft lip is considered a multifactorial defect, resulting from the inter-action between multi-ple genes and various environmental factors.

There is a huge range of these multifactorial conditions, starting with clearly evident defects such as *cleft lip*, in which there is a division in the lip, and *clubfoot*, a deformity in which the foot often has a clublike appearance. Other such abnormalities include congenital heart defects and subtle, long-term problems such as inherited susceptibility to heart disease, diabetes, allergies, and other chronic conditions.

In most cases, detailed knowledge about the causes of these defects is incomplete. It is known that genes are involved because such conditions tend to recur in some families. Yet these birth defects do not follow the pattern of inheritance seen in single-gene defects, making it much more difficult to figure out who in a family will get a multifactorial condition. This is why scientists believe that multiple genes and environmental factors both play a role. The study of these conditions, the environmental factors that are involved, and the gene (or genes) behind them is one of the great frontiers of research in birth defects. The relationship between environment and birth defects will be explored further in Chapters 4, 5, and 6.

CHAPTER 3

CHROMOSOMES AND BIRTH DEFECTS

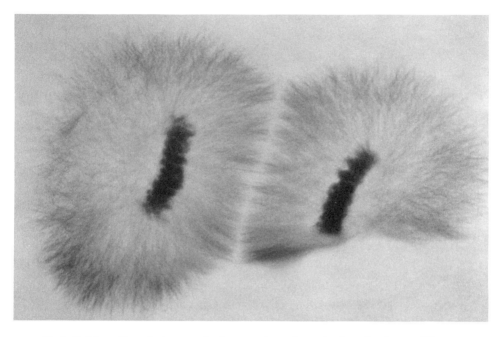

Cell division. The dark area in the center of each developing cell is genetic material.

Sometimes genetic birth defects are not related to mutations in specific genes but instead to problems with the chromosomes themselves. To understand such defects, it is important to know something about cell reproduction.

CELL DIVISION

In order for cells to reproduce themselves, they must divide. Each new cell formed this way contains the identical genetic material as the original. There are two different processes through which this duplication and distribution of genes occurs.

Mitosis

With the exception of the *sex cells*—the male's sperm and the female's eggs—when cells divide they pass on their genetic material through *mitosis*. The process of mitosis and the events leading up to it are as follows:

- **Interphase** In between cell divisions, the nucleus of a cell contains *chromatin*, long, thin fibers made from protein and DNA. Before cell division starts, the DNA in chromatin duplicates itself.

- **Prophase** As division begins, the strands of chromatin coil and condense into rodlike structures used to make the cell's 46 chromosomes. Each chromosome formed is actually made up of two separate strands, called *chromatids*, joined together at an area called the *centromere*. One of these chromatids contains the cell's original DNA, and the other has the duplicate copy, so the two chromatids are actually identical. Also during prophase, two cylindrical bodies in the cell, called *centrioles*, move to opposite sides of the cell. In addition, structures called *microtubules*, which are made from protein, join together to form long *spindle fibers* between the centrioles. The membrane surrounding the cell's nucleus disappears.

- **Metaphase** The chromosomes line up between the centrioles, and spindle fibers become linked to the centromeres.

- **Anaphase** The spindle fibers apparently shorten, pulling the chromosomes apart, with each strand drawn toward the opposite end of the cell.

- **Telophase** The chromosomes elongate back into chromatin, a nuclear envelope forms around the genetic material at each end of the cell, and the spindle fibers vanish.

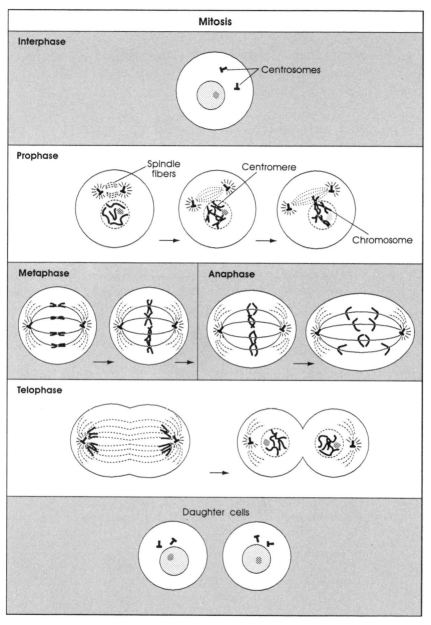

During cell division, a duplicate copy of a cell's genetic material is passed on through mitosis.

When the cell ultimately divides into two, each set of chromatin is trapped in one of the new cells. Thus, each of the newly formed cells contains the same genetic material as the original.

Meiosis

As mentioned, the body's sex cells (also known as *gametes*) do not undergo mitosis. Instead, they receive their genetic material through a more complex process called *meiosis*.

Each sex cell (sperm or egg) contains only one set of chromosomes but is created from a parent cell containing two sets. As the sex cell forms, it undergoes meiosis, during which the genetic material is halved.

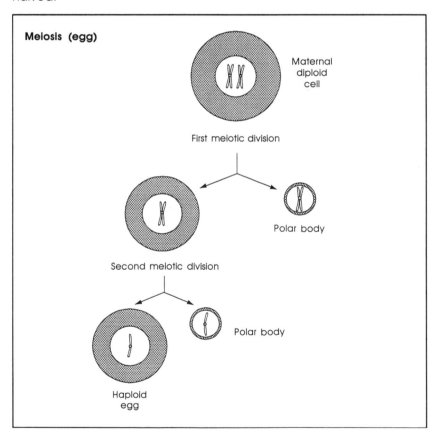

Meiosis (egg)

Maternal diploid cell

First meiotic division

Polar body

Second meiotic division

Polar body

Haploid egg

The sex cells contain only 23 chromosomes, yet are produced from cells containing all 46. The cells used to produce sperm are called *primary spermatocytes*, and those from which the eggs are created are *primary oocytes*. If these parent cells went through ordinary mitosis, the sex cells would also have 46. Meiois, however, leaves them with only half the chromosomes that their parent cells contain.

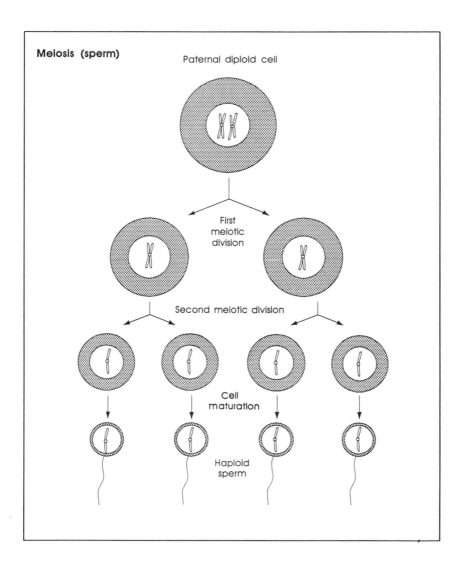

Meiosis (sperm)

Paternal diploid cell

First meiotic division

Second meiotic division

Cell maturation

Haploid sperm

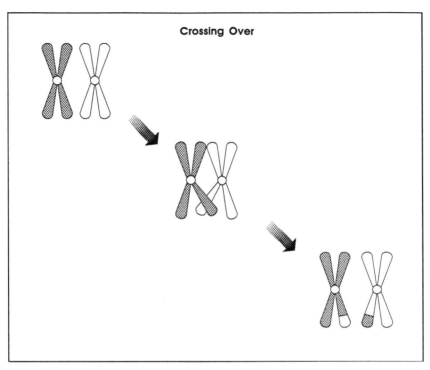

Crossing Over

During the first stage of meiosis, the chromosomes in a pair can become intertwined and exchange sections. In this way, a chromosome may end up with genetic material from both the mother and the father.

The stages of meiosis are somewhat similar to those of mitosis, but there are several differences, including the fact that two separate cell divisions take place instead of one. In the first division, the 23 pairs of chromosomes are divided up, so that just one member of each set is in the newly formed cells. (Cells containing a single set of chromosomes are called *haploid*.) The next division splits up the chromatids, just as in mitosis. In this way, when a sperm fertilizes an egg, the new cells that are formed contain 46 chromosomes, 23 from the father and 23 from the mother. (Cells containing two sets of chromosomes are called *diploid*.) Formation of eggs is called *oogenesis*; creation of sperm cells is *spermatogenesis*. During oogenesis, each cell division produces one large new cell and one smaller *polar body*. The polar bodies have no use and eventually degenerate.

CHROMOSOMAL ERRORS

Of the 23 pairs of chromosomes in a human cell, 22 are listed by number, with chromosome pair 1 the largest and chromosome pair 22 the smallest. The final pair are the sex chromosomes—two X chromosomes for a female, and an X and a Y for a male.

The previous chapter described how alterations in DNA can cause birth defects. But problems can also result from errors in the structure of chromosomes. Often, the effect of a chromosomal error is so severe

After an egg cell and a sperm cell meet, the fertilized egg contains two sets of chromosomes, one from the mother and one from the father.

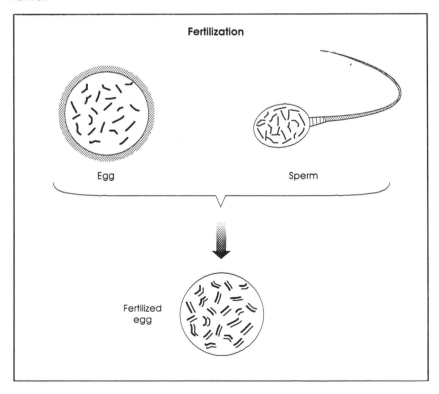

Fertilization

Egg

Sperm

Fertilized egg

that an embryo simply dies. For example, the absence of a single chromosome, a condition called *monosomy*, is almost always lethal. Chromosomal problems, in fact, are believed to occur in 1 of every 13 *conceptions* (the fertilization of an egg by a sperm), with most of these embryos dying soon after fertilization. It is estimated that 60% of the fetuses that are lost by *miscarriage* (in which the woman's body aborts the fetus) in the first three months after conception have a severe chromosome disorder. As a result of this natural elimination, the percentage of fetuses with chromosomal abnormalities drops steadily among women in the later stages of pregnancy. Nevertheless, 1 out of every 125 to 150 newborns has a detectable chromosomal problem. Many defects result from a variety of errors that can occur when chromosomes duplicate or cells divide.

Meiotic Nondisjunction

The most common chromosomal accident is called *meiotic nondis-junction*, which can occur during meiosis. In this error, a pair of chromosome fails to separate, so that one daughter sex cell has no chromosomes from that pair and the other has both. The problem may also occur when the chromosomes separate normally but, in the second half of meiosis, a pair of chromatids does not come apart. In either case, one of the sex cells (egg or sperm) has 24 chromosomes (a condition called *trisomy*) and the other has 22. If fertilization occurs with either of these cells, the result is an abnormal embryo.

Mitotic Nondisjunction

The same sort of error can occur during mitosis early in the life of a normal embryo when it still consists of a small number of cells. In this case, the mistake is called *mitotic nondisjunction*. As a result of this flaw, some of the embryo's cells will be missing one chromosome and others will have an extra chromosome. An individual in whom this occurs will have two populations of cells, a condition called *mosaicism* (although the cells lacking a chromosome tend to die out).

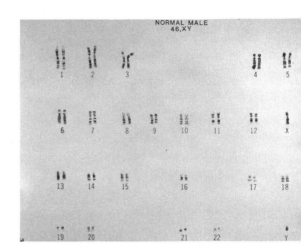

Normal human cells possess 23 pairs of chromosomes. In females, one pair consists of two X chromosomes; males have an X and a Y.

Trisomy Defects

Meiotic nondisjunction is usually the culprit behind Down's syndrome. About 95% of Down's cases are caused by the presence of an extra copy of chromosome 21, a condition called *trisomy 21*. Down's syndrome occurs in 1 out of every 770 live births in the United States. The incidence increases with the age of the mother; although it is not known exactly why, this rise may be due to changes occurring in the mother's eggs as she grows older. The risk is 1 in 250 for a mother age 35, 1 in 69 for a mother age 40, and 1 in 25 for a mother age 46 or older. Down's syndrome is the leading reason for prenatal (before birth) testing, which will be discussed in Chapter 7.

There are a number of other conditions caused by extra chromosomes. These include *trisomy 13* (an extra chromosome 13), also called *Patau's syndrome*, and *trisomy 18*, also known as *Edward's syndrome*. Infants and children with these chromosomal disorders have a variety of physical defects, along with poor mental and physical development. The life spans of these youngsters are short. Children with trisomy 13, for example, suffer from severe mental retardation and have small heads and multiple defects of the eyes, ears, and other organs. They usually die in the first year after birth.

Sex Chromosome Defects

Some conditions are caused by the presence or absence of a sex chromosome. One such disorder is *Turner's syndrome*, which affects 1 out of every 3,500 females born in the United States. A Turner's female has only a single X chromosome. The absence of the other X chromosome does not diminish intelligence, but it can result in a number of abnormalities, including sterility, short stature, a webbed neck, defective hearing, and learning disabilities. The presence of an extra X chromosome in females (their cells contain XXX) occurs in 1 out of every 1,000 births. Some XXX women are normal, but others have mental or reproductive problems and learning disabilities.

A condition caused by the presence of an extra X chromosome in males (so that their cells contain XXY) is *Klinefelter's syndrome*, which affects 1 in 1,000 male babies. Klinfelter's patients tend to be tall and sterile and can suffer from a number of behavioral and psychological problems. In addition, their muscular build can have a feminine appearance, and they may have partially developed breasts.

One genetic type that received an extraordinary amount of attention in the 1960s and 1970s is XYY, the presence of an extra Y chromosome in males. The reason for the publicity was the discovery that more than 3% of males held for crimes against property (which include shoplifting and burglary) in British reform schools were XYY. For a time, it was believed that XYY males were born with a predisposition to violent criminal behavior, but that is no longer thought to be true. Studies have found that although some XYY males are mentally retarded, more than half have normal IQs. They tend to be impulsive and have wild tempers, but the extra Y chromosome does not give them an unusual tendency toward violence. The original misconception probably resulted from the fact that information about XYY males came from studies of men who had gotten into trouble with the law. It is believed, however, that many XYY males lead normal lives.

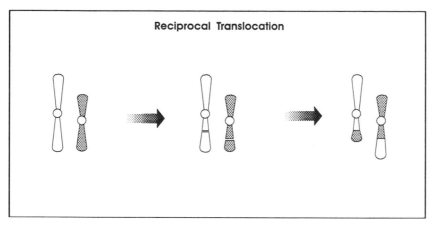

Reciprocal Translocation

Translocation occurs when a piece of chromosome from one pair is replaced with a piece from a member of another pair. In some cases, this can lead to birth defects, such as Down's syndrome.

Fragile X

In the 1970s, Australian researchers discovered a sex chromosome abnormality that now is recognized as the most common inherited cause of mental retardation. It is the *fragile-X syndrome*, and it occurs predominantly in males—about 1 in 1,000. As a result, fragile X is responsible for a quarter of all cases of mental retardation in males.

The syndrome gets its name from the fact that the abnormal X chromosome has a weak spot, giving it a tendency to break. Although fragile X can cause mental retardation ranging from relatively mild to severe, about 20% of males with the condition are of normal intelligence.

But males who are affected by fragile X sometimes have other signs of the condition in combination with mental retardation. These may include a large head with prominent ears and forehead and a large jaw. Other abnormalities can include curvature of the spine and a caved-in breastbone. After puberty, some males with this syndrome have very large testicles. Evidence also suggests that fragile X can, in certain cases, also cause symptoms of *autism*, a condition in which an individual becomes self-absorbed to the point of being closed off from reality.

Two-thirds of females who inherit a fragile X chromosome are of normal intelligence; they are protected by the other, normal X chromosome. About one-third, however, suffer from mental retardation. Some affected females also have the facial characteristics of the syndrome. Recent research has isolated pieces of the fragile X chromosome site. Such studies should help explain the peculiar inheritance patterns of the syndrome.

Deletions and Translocations

Another genetic problem is alteration of the structure of a chromosome. One type of *translocation* occurs when a chromosome from one pair is replaced with a piece from a member of another pair. Translocation does not always lead to abnormal development. Sometimes two chromosomes from different pairs simply exchange pieces (*reciprocal translocation*) to no ill effect. A small percentage of Down's syndrome cases, however, are caused by translocation.

Another abnormality, *deletion*, occurs when a chromosome breaks and a portion of it is lost. For example, a condition called *cri-du-chat* (literally "cry of the cat") *syndrome*, named after the peculiar cry of the affected infant, is caused by a deletion of part of chromosome 5. This error leads to physical defects and, if the child survives, to severe mental retardation.

CHAPTER 4

LIFE-STYLE AND BIRTH DEFECTS

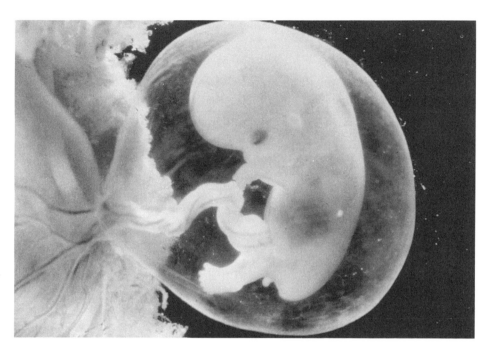

Toxins such as alcohol and nicotine can reach a developing fetus by way of the placenta, the organ through which the child normally receives nourishment. The result can be severe birth defects and miscarriage.

A mother's womb is the environment in which a fetus grows, and so a mother's poor health habits can interfere with a baby's normal development. Several risk factors that can affect a developing fetus have been identified, most notably smoking and drinking.

DRUG-RELATED BIRTH DEFECTS

Alcohol

Consumption of alcohol during pregnancy once was regarded as harmless to the unborn child. Today, concern about the habit has grown so much that all alcoholic beverage bottles contain labels warning women against drinking during pregnancy, and most authorities recommend that a pregnant woman drink no alcohol at all.

A major concern is a condition called *fetal alcohol syndrome*, which was identified in the 1970s. In the United States, 1 out of every 750 babies (about 5,000 per year) is born with this problem. The syndrome is thought to occur primarily in infants whose mothers drink the equivalent of three ounces of pure alcohol every day—the amount of alcohol in six cans of beer or six cocktails.

Babies with fetal alcohol syndrome usually are abnormally small at birth and do not make up the deficit as they get older. Most of them have small, widely spaced eyes; a short, upturned nose; and small, flat cheeks. Defects of the heart and other organs are common. The majority of these infants have smaller than average brains and suffer some degree of mental retardation, along with a short attention span, poor coordination, and behavioral problems. The defects suffered by such children seem to be directly related to the amount of alcohol consumed by their mother. Infants born to mothers who have two to five drinks a day during pregnancy can have some of the physical and mental problems associated with fetal alcohol syndrome, but they tend not to be affected as severely as the children of heavier drinkers.

These problems occur because alcohol passes directly across the *placenta*—the organ through which the fetus receives its nourishment—as soon as the mother has a drink. A fetus is poorly equipped to break down alcohol, so the concentration of alcohol in its blood can actually be higher than the mother's. The precise mechanism by which alcohol harms the fetus is unknown, however, and damage does not seem to be inevitable. Some women who drink heavily during their pregnancy have babies with no signs of fetal alcohol syndrome, where-

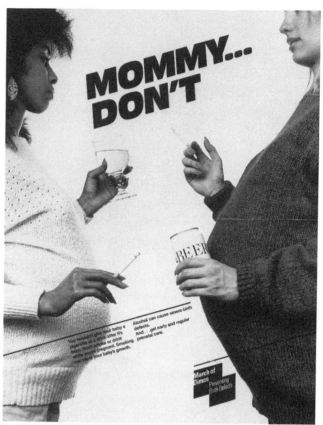

Fetal alcohol syndrome occurs in about 5,000 infants per year in the United States, and all alcoholic beverages now contain labels warning women against drinking during pregnancy.

as infants born to some moderate drinkers have alcohol-related damage. Because there is no way to predict for certain whether a child will be affected, it is best to avoid alcohol completely during pregnancy.

That advice is given even more weight by the fact that alcohol increases the risk of stillbirth and miscarriage. Research indicates that a woman who is a heavy drinker has perhaps twice the normal risk of having a miscarriage.

Cocaine

Cocaine is another drug that can have devastating effects on a fetus. The 1980s saw a substantial increase in the number of pregnant women who used cocaine, often in the deadly form of crack, which is smoked and can cause an immediate, dangerous change in body chemistry.

Women who use cocaine, like those who consume alcohol during pregnancy, are more likely to suffer miscarriage and premature labor. Their babies are at high risk of low birthweight, small head size, stroke, breathing problems, and brain damage. At birth, a cocaine baby goes through something resembling the trauma of withdrawal from the drug, not only becoming irritable and jittery, but crying and jumping at the slightest touch. In addition, these infants do not respond normally to contact by their mother, so that they often fail to form the mother-child bond that is essential for normal emotional development.

Moreover, such babies appear to be more vulnerable to *sudden infant death syndrome*, or SIDS, in which an apparently healthy infant dies in his or her sleep for no known reason. Research suggests that cocaine use among pregnant women doubles the risk of SIDS (although the level of cocaine use that increases the danger is still not known). Even after infancy, cocaine babies may not fully escape the drug's effects. Doctors who are following these children through the early years of life anticipate a higher than normal incidence of learning problems and emotional and developmental difficulties.

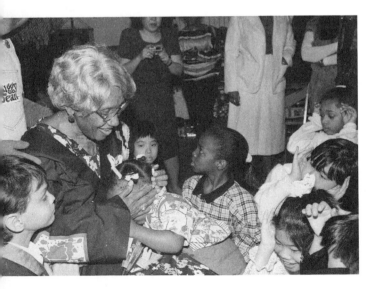

Clara Hale—popularly known as Mother Hale— of New York is well known for her work with children born to mothers who abused drugs during pregnancy. Doctors following the progress of so-called cocaine babies anticipate a higher-than-normal incidence of learning problems and emotional and developmental difficulties among these youngsters.

Marijuana

The hazards of marijuana use during pregnancy are not as clear as with other drugs. A long-term study in Jamaica by Melanie Dreher, dean of the school of nursing at the University of Massachusetts, found that children of Jamaican mothers who smoked marijuana during pregnancy scored higher on developmental tests at the age of one month and at five years than children of nonsmoking mothers. Yet her findings contradict other studies that have related fetal exposure to marijuana with low birthweight, delayed motor development, and other symptoms.

One possible explanation is based on cultural differences. Women in the United States who smoke marijuana are also likely to smoke cigarettes and use other street drugs and alcohol. In Jamaica, marijuana use is more readily accepted as normal behavior and normally is not associated with use of other drugs, including alcohol. Thus, it is possible that the ill effects attributed to marijuana use in the United States actually result from other drugs instead. However, since the research is inconclusive, it should not be assumed that marijuana poses no threat to a fetus.

Good nutrition is only one factor in producing a healthy baby. Steering clear of alcohol, tobacco, and illicit drugs and avoiding exposure to toxins in the workplace are also vitally important.

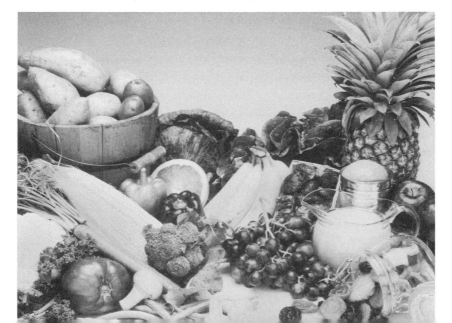

Tobacco

Smoking during pregnancy is another major risk factor for birth defects. Although the mechanism is not exactly clear, research indicates that the damage is done by nicotine, which moves quickly through the placenta, and by a decreased amount of oxygen in the mother's bloodstream, probably due to carbon monoxide in cigarette smoke. (The fetus has been found to have a drastic reduction in breathing movements after its mother smokes two cigarettes.)

Lowering the amount of oxygen in the blood can kill tissue in the placenta. The March of Dimes estimates that smoking is responsible for 20% to 25% of all cases of *placental abruption*, a condition in which the placenta tears away from the wall of the womb, endangering the fetus. The incidence of congenital defects severe enough to cause miscarriage is also increased in smokers. However, damage can be reduced if the mother stops smoking—at best, early in pregnancy, but even in the later stages. It is known that the risk of low birthweight is reduced if a woman gives up cigarettes as late as the last four months of pregnancy.

AGE

Age is another risk factor that requires careful analysis. As mentioned, it has been found that older mothers are at higher risk of bearing a child with Down's syndrome. Results from a recently released Canadian study, however, suggest that when it comes to many other defects, age has no influence. The report looked at 26,859 children born with defects in British Columbia between 1966 and 1981. It excluded babies with Down's syndrome and instances where the mother was known to have taken a medication linked to birth defects, had a family history of genetic disease, was an alcoholic, or had diabetes—a known risk factor for birth defects (see Chapter 5). The study, headed by Dr. Patricia A. Baird, a medical geneticist at the University of British Columbia, concluded that the risk of such defects as cleft palate, spina bifida, cleft lip, congenital heart defects, and limb deformities did not increase with age, even for mothers in their forties.

Indeed, the study found that babies of mothers over age 30 actually had a lower incidence of 3 defects: pyloric stenosis, *patent ductus arteriosis* (a heart condition that causes the blood to circulate incorrectly), and dislocated hip.

FATHERS AND BIRTH DEFECTS

Although the role that a mother's health habits play in birth defects have received widespread attention, until quite recently, male life-style factors were virtually ignored because researchers could not imagine how they would damage sperm. A man typically produces tens of millions of short-lived sperm each day, and it was thought that they were exposed to any toxins in the man's body too briefly to suffer genetic damage. A new theory, however, suggests that toxins can reach the primary spermatocytes. This contact with toxic materials, it is believed, can damage all the sperm produced by a stem cell.

This theory is particularly important because of a growing body of evidence linking birth defects to male exposure to specific toxins. For example, an experiment at the University of Maryland found that when male rats were exposed to relatively low doses of lead, their offspring showed brain abnormalities even though the baby rats' mothers had had no lead exposure. In other studies, male rats that got a third of their

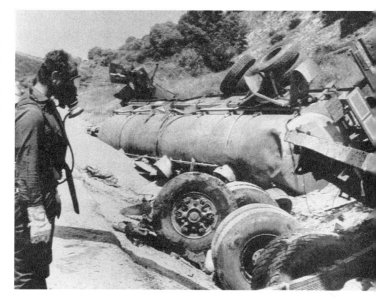

A fireman at the site of a truck wreck in which sulfuric acid was spilled. Previously it was not thought that a male's life-style could cause birth defects. Now, however, it is believed that toxins can affect the stem cells that produce sperm.

calories from alcohol had offspring that displayed learning defects—again, even when the mothers drank no alcohol.

Moreover, research from the University of North Carolina found twice the normal rate of premature births among children of men who work in the glass, clay, stone, textile, and mining industries. The scientists also found evidence that children of male smokers have a higher than normal incidence of brain cancer and leukemia. In addition, research suggests that there is an increased rate of heart defects in children of firemen and an abnormally high rate of cancer and birth defects in the offspring of men who work with spray paints, metal fumes, and certain solvents.

As a result, experts now are giving males the same advice traditionally given to women: If one is planning to have a family, give up smoking, drink moderately (if at all), and try to avoid exposure to toxic substances in the workplace.

A 1991 decision by the Supreme Court gave legal backing to that approach. Johnson Controls, a company that makes automobile batteries, had refused to hire women of childbearing age for jobs that would expose them to lead, an essential ingredient of batteries. The company was sued by the United Auto Workers Union, which charged that the policy was discriminatory. The Supreme Court decided in favor of the union, saying that it was unfair to exclude women but not men from jobs that expose them to toxic substances. In making its decision, the court rejected the Johnson contention that men are less likely than women to cause birth defects. The implications of the court decision and of research on the male role in birth defects are just beginning to be examined.

CHAPTER 5

DISEASE, CHEMICALS, AND RADIATION

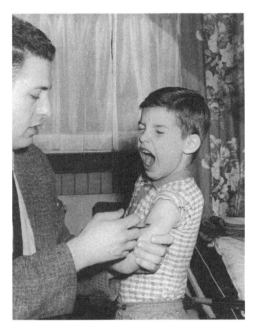

Vaccination against childhood disease is not always a pleasant experience—as this 1961 photo attests. The rubella vaccine has proved essential against both disease and birth defects.

INFECTION AND BIRTH DEFECTS

When a pregnant woman contracts an infection, disease microorganisms can enter the fetus's bloodstream through the placenta. In other cases, the baby may be exposed to the disease in the birth canal during delivery. Unfortunately, a number of infections are known to increase the risk of birth defects. One of the most clear-cut examples is *German measles*, or *rubella*. Although symptoms of the disease are relatively mild, rubella can be devastating to a fetus if the mother contracts it during pregnancy, especially in the first three months. According to the American College of Obstetricians and Gynecologists, 50% of the children born to women who contract German measles in the first four weeks of pregnancy have birth defects. The rate declines during the course of pregnancy, however, dropping to 10% by the third month.

The disease causes a distinctive pattern of defects called *congenital rubella syndrome*, which can include *cataracts* (in which the lens of the eye becomes cloudy) and other eye problems; abnormalities of the major blood vessels of the heart; deafness; delayed language development; mental retardation and an abnormally small brain; and a multitude of other defects affecting the skin, bones, lungs, and other organs.

A vaccine against German measles was approved by the U.S. Food and Drug Administration in 1969, shortly after a major epidemic that led to the birth of more than 20,000 children in the United States with congenital rubella syndrome. The vaccine has dramatically reduced the

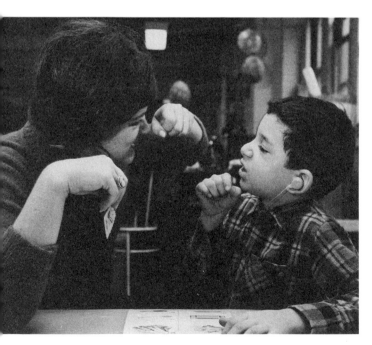

A child suffering from rubella-related birth defects undergoes therapy. Congenital rubella syndrome can affect the eyes and heart and result in deafness and mental retardation.

incidence of the syndrome and is recommended for all women before pregnancy. However, women of childbearing age who did not get the vaccine when they were younger should be vaccinated only if they are certain they are not pregnant and do not expect to be pregnant in the next three months. Although no birth defects have been reported in children of women who were immunized during pregnancy, there is a small risk that problems could occur, since the vaccine contains the virus itself.

Cytomegalovirus

Another infection that can lead to birth defects is caused by *cytomegalovirus* (CMV), a type of herpesvirus. It is widespread; about half the American population is infected with CMV by the age of 30. The infection, which can be spread through sexual or nonsexual contact, usually goes unnoticed and does no damage, although it can cause symptoms resembling those of the common cold. In addition, the majority of infants born to women infected with the virus apparently suffer no ill effects from it. The chance of birth defects seems particularly low if the mother is first infected before she becomes pregnant. However, research indicates that if a woman who has never before been infected with CMV gets it during the first half of her pregnancy, she runs a much greater risk of having an infant with significant problems. Part of the reason may be that the mother does not have the chance to build up any disease-fighting antibodies against the virus to protect both herself and her fetus. Defects caused by CMV include impaired hearing, seizures, blindness, and mental retardation. Learning disabilities also occur. It is believed that in the United States up to 10,000 children per year suffer defects that are caused by congenital CMV infection.

Blood tests to detect cytomegalovirus are recommended for pregnant women who show signs of the infection. Neither a vaccine nor an effective drug is available, however, but pregnant women are advised to follow the rules of good hygiene to limit the risk of infection, which usually occurs on exposure to contaminated saliva, blood, or other body fluids.

Chicken Pox

Infection with *chicken pox* (caused by another type of herpesvirus) can also cause birth defects if it is contracted early in pregnancy. The risk is relatively small, however, because 95% of American adults have already been infected as children, making them immune to a second bout with the disease. The incidence of *congenital chicken pox syndrome* is very low, but when it does occur, damage can include muscle and bone defects, mental retardation, blindness, and seizures. A pregnant woman who has not previously had chicken pox should limit her exposure to young children because the disease is so prevalent in youngsters. If a woman is exposed to chicken pox during pregnancy, injections of *gamma globulin* (a type of blood protein) can prevent the disease. A chicken pox vaccine was in an advanced state of development in 1991 and is expected to be available soon.

Toxoplasmosis

Toxoplasmosis, caused by a protozoon that often infects cats and is found in raw meat, is a serious threat during pregnancy. A baby that was infected with toxoplasmosis in the womb can later suffer an acute

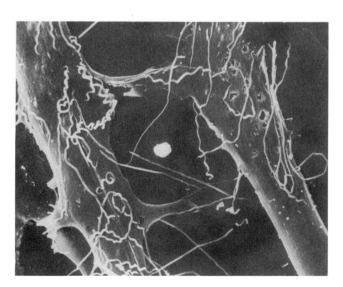

Sexually transmitted disease can have devastating effects on an unborn child. Syphilis, caused by the bacteria Treponema pallidum (seen in this microscopic view), can result in mental retardation, blindness, paralysis, and other severe defects.

(severe, short-term) illness, with fever and convulsions. In addition, the infection can result in stillbirth, miscarriage, or severe birth defects, including mental retardation, visual and hearing impairment, and learning disorders.

A woman should be tested for toxoplasmosis early in pregnancy. If she has been previously infected, there is no danger to her fetus because she has already built up an immunity against future infections. If she has not been infected, however, she should avoid eating raw or undercooked meat and should also avoid exposure to cats. A cat's litter box should be cleaned every day, but not by the pregnant woman. Since toxoplasmosis spores can survive in soil, an expectant mother should wear gloves while gardening.

Sexually Transmitted Diseases

Sexually transmitted diseases are another source of birth defects. *Syphilis*, for example, can be passed through the mother to her unborn child. This *prenatal syphilis* can cause damage to the central nervous system, blindness, paralysis, and other devastating abnormalities.

Genital herpes, which affects at least 5 million Americans, can also cause birth defects. The disease can result in repeated outbreaks of painful sores in the genital area. If an infected woman delivers a baby during such an outbreak, the infant can come in contact with the virus as he or she passes through the birth canal. This exposure proves fatal in about half the cases. Of those infants who survive, half of them suffer permanent damage to the nervous system. However a doctor can protect a baby from the virus by performing a *cesarean section*, a surgical procedure in which the child is delivered through an incision in the abdomen.

DIABETES

Diabetes requires extremely careful handling during pregnancy. The incidence of major birth defects in infants born to women with diabetes is two to three times higher than for nondiabetics. The reason is that high levels of blood sugar found in diabetics somehow affect the normal development of the fetus in the first weeks of pregnancy. Among the defects that can occur is *macrosomia*, in which the newborn has an abnormally large body size.

Such problems need not occur, however. Several studies have shown that strict control of blood sugar levels before and during pregnancy can protect the fetus from harm. For example, a 1991 study at the University of California at San Francisco compared 194 diabetic women. Eighty-four of them were coached on blood sugar control methods and diet before they became pregnant. The other 110 women received the same help, but only after their pregnancies began. Only one child with a major birth defect was born to the women who received

The herbicide Agent Orange is sprayed by U.S. forces over an enemy position in Vietnam. Veterans of that war maintain that exposure to Agent Orange is responsible for birth defects in their children.

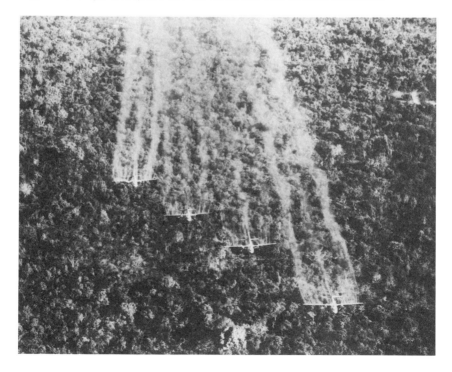

the prepregnancy coaching. However, 12 major birth defects occurred in the babies whose diabetic mothers started strict control methods during pregnancy.

TOXINS AND BIRTH DEFECTS

The question of a link between toxic chemicals and birth defects is a controversial one because it usually is difficult to prove such a connection. There are some exceptions, however. Mercury poisoning is known to be a major danger to the developing fetus. The most horrendous example occurred in the Minimata region of Japan, where an industrial company dumped large amounts of mercury-containing wastes into the sea near a fishing village. Fish in the sea were contaminated by the mercury, and women who ate the fish bore children with severe brain damage and crippling limb abnormalities. The Minimata tragedy continued for many years, until blame was finally fixed on mercury and the company acknowledged responsibility. Exposure to smaller amounts of mercury can cause more subtle brain and nerve defects, so pregnant women are told to avoid fish contaminated with even very low concentrations of industrial mercury.

Exposure to lead also is clearly linked to neurological and kidney problems. Lead affects the nervous system so severely that subtle defects in IQ and other mental functions have been found in children with blood levels of lead that once were regarded as safe. Those studies were a primary reason for legislation banning the use of lead in gasoline.

But the case against many other suspected toxins is not as clear. One example is the ongoing debate about the effects of *Agent Orange*, the herbicide sprayed on vegetation by the U.S. military during the Vietnam War. Agent Orange contains trace amounts of *dioxin*, a chemical suspected of causing cancer and birth defects. Veterans of Vietnam maintain that exposure to Agent Orange is responsible for many birth defects among their children. Scientific studies have produced no clear-cut evidence for or against dioxin as a birth defect risk. Some studies have found an association, whereas others have not, so questions about dioxin remain.

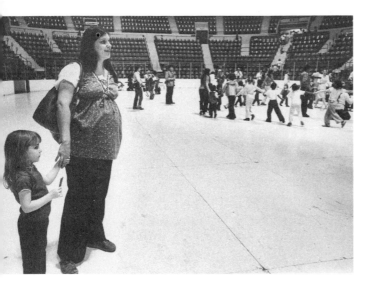

Radiation is another potential source of birth defects. In 1979, radiation released during an accident at Pennsylvania's Three Mile Island nuclear power plant forced pregnant women and young children to this evacuation center.

The situation regarding the toxic waste dumped at the Love Canal area near Niagara Falls in New York is similar. Between 1942 and 1953, a chemical company dumped about 22,000 tons of toxic chemical wastes into a hole that had originally been dug for a canal near Niagara Falls, New York. The site was covered over in 1953 and homes later sprang up in the area. By 1977, however, chemicals were leaking from the rotting steel drums into local storm sewers, gardens, and basements. In addition, residents claimed that there was an unusually high rate of birth defects, miscarriages, cancers, and other health problems in their community. Hundreds of families in the vicinity were eventually relocated by the state and federal governments, but there is still no solid scientific evidence for increased birth defects among the offspring of women who lived near Love Canal.

In case after case, it has proved equally difficult to show clear links between environmental exposures to toxic materials and birth defects as it has been to show no connections. What can be said is that a number of industrial, business, and household chemicals have been identified as possible causes of birth defects. These include *poly-chlorinated biphenyls*, or PCBs, which have been phased out as insulating material because of their potential danger to the unborn; pesticides; certain solvents; toluene (which is used in industrial cleansers); and hair dyes. In almost every case, there are studies that have produced opposing results, some showing danger and some showing none.

RADIATION AND BIRTH DEFECTS

Whether radiation emitted by computer *video display terminals*, or VDTs, poses a danger also remains uncertain. This is an important question, considering the huge number of offices now using computers for word processing and other jobs. There have been reports of an increased number of miscarriages and birth defects for women working with VDTs. A study in the late 1980s by Dr. Kelly Ann Brix of the University of Michigan found a slight increase in miscarriages for women who used VDTs for more than 20 hours a week, but the

Even a seemingly harmless video display terminal may be cause for concern among pregnant women. Although a recent study found no increased risk of birth defects among babies born to women exposed to VDT radiation, research into the question continues.

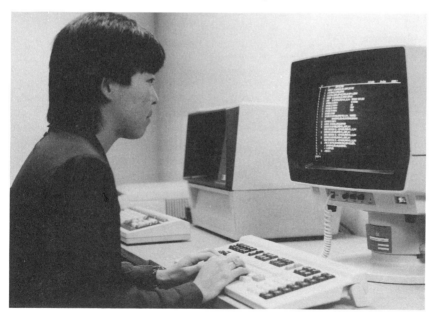

results were inconclusive because only a small number of pregnancies was examined.

A more conclusive study was reported in March 1991 by researchers at the National Institute of Occupational Safety and Health. They looked at 2,430 women over a 6-year period and reported that there was "no difference in risk" of miscarriage, birth defects, and other birth-related problems between those who sat in front of a VDT for more than 25 hours a week and those in comparable jobs who did not not use video terminals. The report provided what seemed to be authoritative reassurance about VDTs and birth defects, but other studies are continuing.

X rays are another source of concern. It has been found, for example, that exposing a fetus to X rays, especially early in pregnancy, can cause *microcephaly* (in which the head is abnormally small) and mental retardation, eye and bone abnormalities, and cleft palate. Most of those problems, however, occur only if the fetus is exposed to high levels of radiation, levels used for treatment of conditions such as cancer, rather than the smaller X-ray doses used for diagnosing broken bones. This fact is reassuring for women who may have diagnostic X-ray exposure before they realize they are pregnant. Research suggests, however, that there may be a link between even relatively small amounts of X-ray exposure in the womb and increased incidence of childhood leukemia. Therefore, women attempting to become pregnant are advised to avoid any unnecessary medical radiation.

CHAPTER 6

MEDICINES AND BIRTH DEFECTS

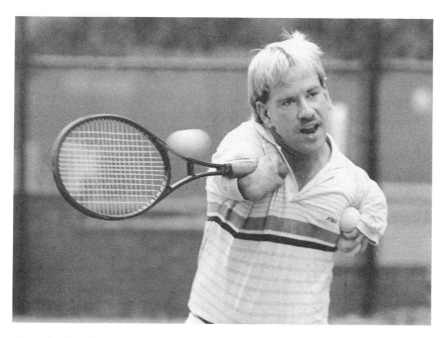

Despite hand and arm deformities caused by the medication thalidomide, this man overcame his birth defects to become an instructor at a Georgia tennis club.

The dangers of taking medications during pregnancy became dramatically clear in the 1960s, when women in Europe began giving birth to children with catastrophic deformities of the arms and legs and other severe birth defects. The blame eventually was traced to thalidomide, a medication that was being prescribed for nausea during pregnancy. Thalidomide had caused no defects in animal tests, but it had a devastating impact on children whose mothers took it early in pregnancy. Fortunately for American women, the drug was not marketed in the

United States because an alert physician at the Food and Drug Administration held back approval while she checked out reports that thalidomide might be dangerous.

PRESCRIPTION DRUGS

Accutane

To date, however, only a small number of prescription drugs are known for certain to cause birth defects if taken during pregnancy. The clearest example is *Accutane*, a synthetic vitamin A compound that is prescribed for an extremely severe and disfiguring type of acne. Accutane, like other forms of vitamin A, has been known for many years to cause a variety of birth defects, including facial deformities, heart defects, mental retardation, and abnormalities of the central nervous system. When federal officials approved the marketing of Accutane, they required a label on the package warning against the drug's use by women who may become pregnant while taking it. In addition, doctors are told to perform a pregnancy test before prescribing the medication for any woman of childbearing age. Yet it has been impossible to eliminate Accutane-caused birth defects completely. Critics have demanded that Accutane be taken off the market, but it remains in use because it is the only available treatment for a serious condition.

Anticonvulsant Drugs

Several drugs for epilepsy, called *anticonvulsants* because they prevent or relieve convulsions, are also associated with an increased risk of birth defects. A woman taking one of a group of anticonvulsants known as *phenytoins* during pregnancy runs two to three times the normal risk of bearing a child with a defect such as cleft lip or cleft palate or with deformed genitals or kidneys. Another anticonvulsant, *valproic acid*, is associated with an increased incidence of spina bifida. However, the risk associated with anticonvulsant drugs is not entirely clear because it is possible that the epilepsy itself is a contributing factor for birth defects. At any rate, the question poses a dilemma for women with this disease as well as for their physicians. The decision to continue taking anticonvulsant drugs ideally is made by both, after a serious discussion. In many cases, the risk to the fetus is great even if medication is discontinued because convulsions can endanger both mother and unborn child.

Sex Hormones

Sex hormones, specifically the synthetic hormone *diethystilbestrol*, or DES, can cause birth defects. DES was widely prescribed during the 1960s under the mistaken belief that it helped to prevent miscarriage. Its use was discontinued when studies showed it had no beneficial effect, but not before tens of thousands of fetuses had been exposed to it. Female children exposed to DES in the womb can have abnormalities of the genital tract. They also run a slightly increased risk of genital cancer later in life. (In addition, some male children have been

Sex hormones taken by pregnant women have been known to cause birth defects; the drug DES caused abnormalities of the genital tract among females exposed to it in the womb. Oral contraceptives are another source of sex hormones, although they are not thought to pose a high risk of defects.

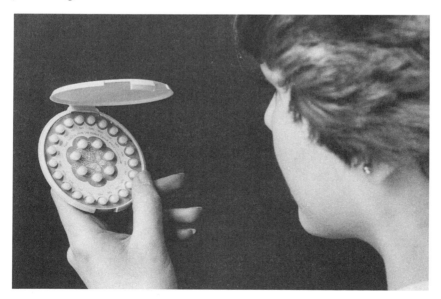

found to have abnormalities of the urogenital tract.) Another possible source of exposure to sex hormones is the birth control pill. However, women who take oral contraceptives during pregnancy (because they do not yet know they are pregnant) run a relatively low risk of hormone-related defects.

Anticoagulants

Warfarin, an *anticoagulant* (a drug that reduces blood clotting), can harm a fetus's bones and cartilage, result in blindness and mental retardation, or cause stillbirth and miscarriage. This drug is prescribed to prevent *thrombosis*, the formation of clots that block arteries and veins. As in the case of anticonvulsants, the decision to use anticoagulants during pregnancy depends on the mother's medical condition.

Antibiotics

Most antibiotics appear to be safe to use during pregnancy, but there are exceptions. Exposure in the womb to some members of the *tetracycline* group can cause permanent staining of a child's first set of teeth. *Streptomycin*, which is used to treat tuberculosis, can cause deafness through nerve damage.

Other Drugs

The list of other medications that are known to cause birth defects is rather short and includes mostly drugs for conditions that are uncommon during pregnancy—for example, anticancer drugs, whose function is to kill cells, and *penicillamine*, a compound used to prevent the excess buildup of copper in the body that occurs in a rare genetic condition called *Wilson's disease*. The list of drugs about which doubts have been expressed or about which little is known is longer.

One prime example is *Bendectin*, a medicine that was taken by millions of pregnant women in the United States to control the severe

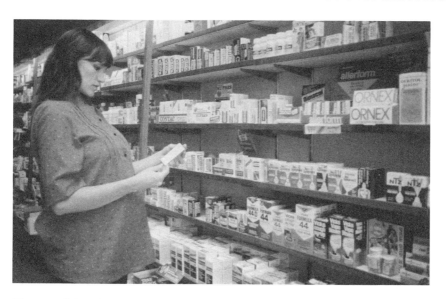

The possible effects that medicines may have on a developing fetus are of particular concern, considering that women in the United States may take anywhere from 4 to 14 prescription and nonprescription drugs over the course of a pregnancy.

nausea and morning sickness that are common early in pregnancy. There were several reports in the 1970s and 1980s that Bendectin was responsible for a small number of limb and heart defects in fetuses. Scientific studies failed to prove these assertions, but so many lawsuits were filed that the company that marketed the drug withdrew it from sale in 1983, saying that legal costs were too high. Supporters of Bendectin argue that the drug is less dangerous to the fetus than the vomiting and nausea it can prevent, but the medication remains off the market. Similarly, there has been suspicion that some tranquilizers can cause birth defects, but the evidence is inconclusive.

The standard advice now given to pregnant women is to avoid all drugs, especially early in pregnancy and even during the period when a woman is trying to become pregnant. If a medicine must be taken, its safety should be checked beforehand with a physician. In an area where there are great uncertainties, the wisest course is to avoid any conceivable risk, if possible.

NONPRESCRIPTION DRUGS

The number of drugs known to cause birth defects is small, yet there are continuing concerns about the effects of medications taken during pregnancy. One reason for this is that pregnant women in the United States take a large number of drugs—anywhere from 4 to 14 over the course of the pregnancy, according to several surveys. Some of these are prescription medications that must be taken for specific medical conditions, but others are over-the-counter products that women do not hesitate to use because they are not perceived as drugs. For example, few women worry about taking aspirin for a headache, yet aspirin is known to reduce blood clotting, which in turn could lead to excess bleeding.

Concern extends beyond medications. Few people regard having a cup of coffee or drinking a cola as drug taking, yet coffee and cola drinks contain caffeine. One study, in which mice were given what would have amounted to about 12 to 24 cups of coffee per day in a human, provided some evidence that caffeine could lead to defects. Since then, however, research has not shown that this is true of normal coffee consumption. The U.S. Food and Drug Administration advises pregnant women to limit the amount of caffeine they consume. Doctors also worry about the interaction of drugs with each other and with other chemicals. In animal tests, for example, the frequency of birth defects is increased if rats are given aspirin together with *benzoic acid*, a common food preservative. Considering the widespread use of chemicals in modern society, the number of possible interactions is virtually limitless.

CHAPTER 7

PRENATAL DETECTION AND TREATMENT

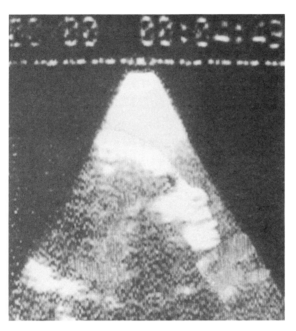

*Ultrasound image of a fetus. During amnio-
centesis, sound waves are used to produce
an image of the unborn child, so that the
needle can be safely inserted.*

It is possible to detect an increasing number of birth defects and genetic diseases in the womb. In rare cases, defects have even been repaired before birth. The field of prenatal detection and treatment is still growing and developing, but its roots go back more than half a century.

In the 1930s, doctors found that they could safely insert a needle into the womb and remove a sample of the *amniotic fluid*, the protective fluid that surrounds the fetus in the womb. In the early 1960s, this technique, called *amniocentesis*, was used to make the first prenatal diagnosis of a condition that can threaten a fetus, *Rh blood group incompatibility*.

Rh FACTOR

About 85% of white Americans and 99% of blacks have a specific substance on the surface of their blood cells called the *Rh factor*, so called because it was first found in rhesus monkeys. People with the factor are said to be *Rh positive*, and those without it are *Rh negative*. If Rh-positive blood is given to an Rh-negative person, the Rh-positive red cells are identified by the immune system as foreign invaders and are attacked and destroyed.

Trouble can occur when an Rh-negative woman becomes pregnant by an Rh-positive man. If the fetus is Rh-positive, the mother's immune system may attack the red blood cells of the fetus, damaging or killing the unborn child. As a result, in the 1960s doctors began analyzing samples of amniotic fluid to determine whether Rh incompatibility existed in a given pregnancy. (Today physicians can make the diagnosis using another method: removing a sample of fetal blood from the umbilical cord.)

Normally, a problem does not occur with the first Rh-positive baby because the mother's immune system has not yet built up a defense against the infant's blood. But difficulties arise if a subsequent child is Rh positive because then the woman's immune system is ready to attack. However, the condition is often treated by injecting the mother with a serum that prevents her from building a defense against the Rh factor. One of the major implications of progress against Rh incompatibility was the demonstration that diagnosis and treatment of fetal problems was possible, something once regarded as beyond the reach of medicine.

SEX DETERMINATION

Another advance occurred in the 1950s, when two Canadian doctors, M. L. Barr and E. G. Bertram, discovered that it was possible to determine the sex of an unborn baby by examining the fetal cells found in the amniotic fluid. They found that cells of female babies, but not males, had a distinctive dark area, called the *Barr body*. This discovery was employed in the 1960s to help parents determine whether a fetus was at risk of having a sex-linked genetic disorder.

Moreover, as the science of genetics developed, so did prenatal detection of birth defects. By the mid-1960s, new techniques allowed scientists to grow cells in the lab taken from amniotic fluid. The chromosomes of those cells could then be examined for abnormalities. In 1968, the first prenatal detection of Down's syndrome was performed this way by Dr. Carlo Valenti in New York City.

TESTING FOR DEFECTS

Amniocentesis

Amniocentesis allows physicians to diagnose many conditions prenatally. The procedure usually is done between the 14th and 16th weeks

Amniocentesis can be used to test for dozens of fetal birth defects. A hollow needle is inserted through the mother's abdominal wall into the womb, and a sample of amniotic fluid is removed. The fetal cells are then separated out and allowed to multiply in the lab, where their genetic material can be analyzed.

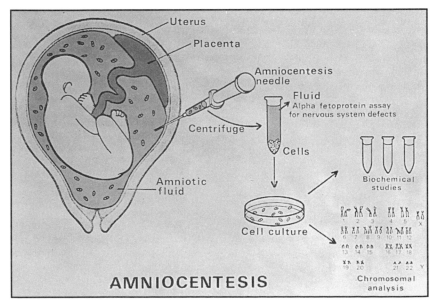

AMNIOCENTESIS

of pregnancy. The obstetrician performs amniocentesis by inserting a thin needle into the womb, commonly using *ultrasound*—a method that bounces sound waves off objects to form a picture of them—to get an image of the fetus and thus prevent the needle from harming it. Fetal cells are removed from the amniotic fluid sample and are grown for two to three weeks. By then they have multiplied so that there are enough of them to allow their analysis. Amniocentesis carries a very small risk of miscarriage—about 1 in 300 to 400, according to most studies. This danger must be balanced against the risk of bearing a child suffering from a serious defect.

Chorionic Villi Sampling

A newer technique called *chorionic villi sampling*, which allows testing much earlier in pregnancy, came into use in the United States during

Using amniocentesis, doctors are able to test for Rh blood group incompatibility, so named because the Rh factor was first found in rhesus monkeys.

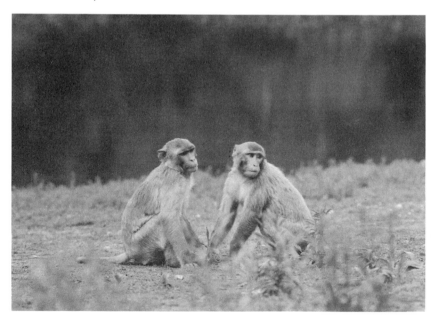

the 1980s. In one version of this procedure, the obstetrician passes a thin plastic tube called a *catheter* through the vagina and uses suction to remove a small sample of the tiny fingerlike projections called *villi* that extend from the *chorion*, the membrane surrounding the fetus. The chorionic cells in this sample have the identical genetic makeup of the fetus. The procedure can be performed as early as the ninth week of pregnancy.

The safety of chorionic villi sampling has been an issue since the technique was introduced. There is a slight risk of infection and of vaginal bleeding, and some studies have also shown a miscarriage rate greater than 2%. However, that figure could be misleading because women normally have a relatively high rate of miscarriage early in pregnancy. That makes it difficult to know how often the test itself is responsible. The latest statistics gathered by the National Institutes of Health (NIH), which compared 2,278 women who had chorionic villi sampling and 671 who had amniocentesis, found no difference in the percentage of miscarriages.

MSAFP

Another form of prenatal testing that has become common is a blood test called the *maternal serum alpha-fetoprotein screening test*, or MSAFP. This examination is performed in the 16th to 18th week of pregnancy. The doctor takes a sample of the mother's blood and tests it for a substance called *alpha-fetoprotein*, or AFP, which the fetus makes in large amounts during the first three months of pregnancy. Some AFP gets into the amniotic fluid, and a smaller amount escapes into the mother's bloodstream.

Some fetal abnormalities cause large amounts of AFP to reach the mother's blood. Neural tube defects, for example, such as spina bifida and anencephaly, create openings through which excessive amounts of AFP reach the mother. Other disorders have the same effect. One of them is *omphalocele*, which exposes the intestines of the fetus. More-over, for unknown reasons, large amounts of AFP are released in high-risk pregnancies in which the fetus is in danger of stillbirth, low birthweight, or premature delivery. A very low level of AFP indicates other problems, including Down's syndrome, trisomy 13, and trisomy 18 (although decreased AFP will not always result from these conditions).

Although the MSAFP test can suggest the possibility of a defect, it cannot be used to show exactly which problem exists or to prove whether there is a defect at all. According to the American College of Obstetricians and Gynecologists (ACOG), of every 1,000 women tested, about 50 will have AFP levels above the normal range. Often, however, these readings indicate only that the dating of the pregnancy is wrong. Maternal blood levels of AFP rise steadily until the 28th or 32nd week of pregnancy. A level that is normal for the 16th week of pregnancy is read as abnormal for the 18th week. An ultrasound examination can be used to determine the age of the fetus and discover whether the AFP level is truly abnormal.

Of the 50 women with high AFP levels, according to the ACOG, 10 to 15 are further along in the pregnancy than had been thought; 3 to 8 are carrying more than 1 fetus (twins and triplets release more AFP than a single child); and 5 have an increased chance of miscarriage. Only 1 or 2 of the others will be found to be carrying a fetus suffering from a neural tube defect. Both ultrasound and amniocentesis are used to make these diagnoses. If no obvious reason for excess AFP is found, an expectant mother will be monitored carefully because her fetus may be at high risk of stillbirth or low birthweight, or the mother may have an increased chance of going into labor too early. Experience has shown, however, that the majority of these pregnancies end safely.

Even though it is far from perfect, the MSAFP test is recommended for all pregnancies. California law requires obstetricians to offer the test to every pregnant woman; a woman who declines the test must sign a form. Nevertheless, the MSAFP exam, like all other prenatal tests, is performed only with the pregnant woman's consent.

Recently some centers have begun to test not only for AFP but for two hormones as well: *human chorionic gonadotropin*—a high level of which indicates Down's syndrome—and *unconjugated estriol*—a low level of which can also suggest a defect. If the test results are abnormal, an ultrasound examination and amniocentesis can be done to make a diagnosis.

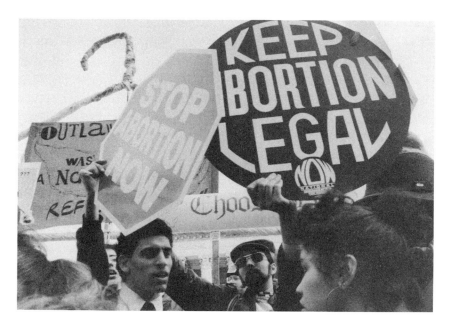

The medical community's ability to test for birth defects has contributed to difficult ethical questions. Some people believe that a parent deserves the right to choose whether to bring a handicapped child into the world or to terminate a pregnancy through abortion. Others believe that no fetus should be terminated before birth.

ETHICAL ISSUES AND GENETIC COUNSELING

All prenatal tests raise serious issues of ethics and morality. Prenatal testing cannot be done in a psychological vacuum. It is one thing to know the abstract fact that each person carries a certain number of potentially harmful recessive genes. It is quite another for two people to learn that they carry such a gene and that their unborn child is at risk of a serious birth defect or death because of this. Inevitably, many parents have feelings of guilt and self-doubt when they are told of the problem. To meet the emotional needs of people facing such a situation, a new discipline called *genetic counseling* has been developed.

Genetic counseling is normally performed by a physician or by a specially trained counselor. It is intended for people who have a genetic disease, who carry the gene for one, or who are otherwise at high risk of bearing an affected baby. The purpose of genetic counseling is to explain the odds that a couple faces of having a child who suffers from a defect and to discuss treatment options for a specific condition.

The ideal counselor is familiar not only with genetic diseases and other birth defects but also with human nature. Experience has shown that information about genetic risk often is misinterpreted and that various factors, including anxiety and other emotions, can complicate the choice a couple must make.

Sometimes a couple must decide whether to continue a pregnancy in which the fetus is known to have a defect or whether to terminate the pregnancy through abortion. Fortunately the great majority of prenatal diagnoses—perhaps 97%—reveal that the fetus is normal. In the other 3% of cases, however, parents must determine whether they—and society—can bear the burden of caring for a child with a defect. Genetic counselors know that these decisions are highly individual.

Opponents of abortion say that no fetus, however painful and short its future life will be, should be terminated before birth. Those on the other side of the issue maintain that a woman should have the right to choose whether to bring a handicapped infant into the world because some parents may consider it unfair and cruel to permit the pain and suffering of a child destined to be born with a severe defect.

CHAPTER 8

FRONTIERS

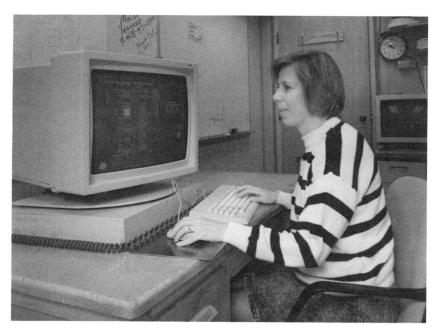

Researchers on the Human Genome Project are engaged in a 15-year effort to find the correct sequence of the 3 billion base pairs that make up humankind's genes. If successful, scientists expect to gain far greater understanding of genetic birth defects.

A NEW ERA

On September 14, 1990, a team of physicians at the National Institutes of Health made medical history. They gave a four-year-old girl from Texas a transfusion of her own blood cells that had been changed by genetic engineering. It was the opening of an era of human gene therapy.

The girl was born with a condition that prevented her from producing an enzyme called *adenosine deaminase*, or ADA. Without it, her body's immune system could not develop properly. Even the slightest infection would threaten her life, and she was forced to live in an isolated, germ-free environment. The NIH team, led by Drs. Steven A. Rosenberg, W. French Anderson, and R. Michael Blaese, altered her blood cells by inserting the gene for ADA production. Months later, they reported that the altered cells were providing at least some of the ADA that the child's body could not previously make.

Gene therapy has been made possible by a series of rapid advances in genetics. These new findings now permit molecular biologists to isolate and learn the nature of the genes responsible for many diseases.

Drs. Steven A. Rosenberg (left) and R. Michael Blaese of the National Institutes of Health helped to open the door to a new era in medicine. They inserted genetically altered blood cells into a youngster suffering from a dangerous enzyme deficiency, so that her body could manufacture the needed substance.

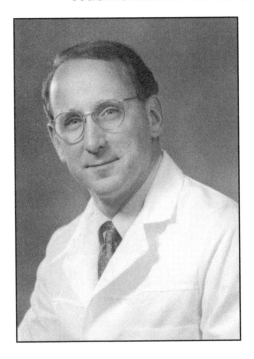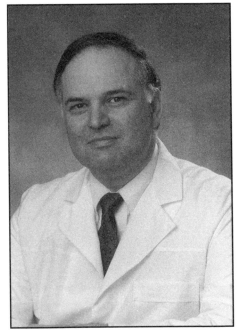

In the past few years, research teams have isolated the genes for cystic fibrosis, muscular dystrophy, and retinoblastoma. The search for many other such genes is underway, and one effort, the Human Genome Project, offers particular hope.

THE HUMAN GENOME PROJECT

A 15-year program to find all the genes in the human body officially began in 1990. Organized by the National Institutes of Health and the U.S. Department of Energy, the Human Genome Project is being carried out in laboratories across the United States and abroad. The ultimate goal of the program is to find the correct sequence of the 3 billion base pairs that make up humankind's genes. One result, scientists believe, will be the discovery of the mutated genes behind thousands of genetic birth defects. The portion of the work being carried out in the United States alone may cost as much as $3 billion.

GENE THERAPY

Identifying the genes responsible for birth defects will open the way to gene therapy for many such conditions. Using specially altered viruses, molecular biologists can insert working genes into human cells to do the work of mutated genes.

Although the technology for gene therapy now exists, much developmental work is needed. Many genetic conditions affect only certain tissues—muscular dystrophy, for example, causes wasting of the muscles. To repair the damage, it is necessary to get genetically altered cells to the appropriate tissues. Experiments to that end are proceeding using animals or utilizing cells grown in the laboratory.

Cell Implantation

In theory—and as laboratory experiments increasingly suggest—it is possible to diagnose and treat some conditions before birth by genetic therapy that implants healthy cells in a fetus. Taking biomedical technology one step further, an even more daring technique could be possible for couples known to carry genes for a potentially fatal condition. An egg could be fertilized in the laboratory and tested for the presence of the mutated gene. The condition could then be corrected by inserting the nonmutated gene in the embryo, which would then be implanted in the womb for a normal pregnancy.

Ethical Issues of Gene Therapy

There is currently an intense debate about the ethical and moral nature of this sort of gene therapy. On one side are those who say there is no reason why biomedical technology should not be used to relieve the human suffering caused by genetic disease. On the other side are those

Doctors examine the results of an amniocentesis test. New insight into birth defects is opening the way for gene therapy through which physicians may one day cure previously hopeless conditions by attacking them on a genetic level.

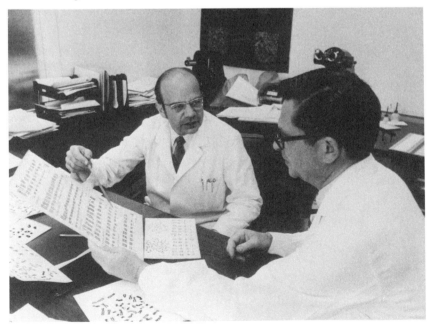

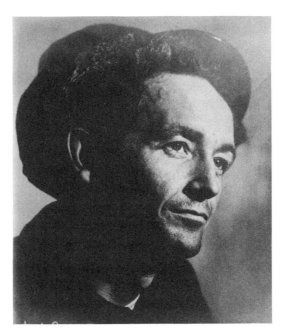

Folksinger Woody Guthrie fell victim to the fatal condition known as Huntington's chorea. Medicine's increasing ability to identify people with incurable genetic defects will undoubtedly raise many new ethical questions concerning a patient's right to know about his or her health.

who consider it ethically unacceptable to alter the very nature of a human embryo. The debate continues, and it will become sharper as the technology of gene therapy improves.

OTHER QUESTIONS

There are additional ethical issues posed by advances in medical science. Another question concerns identification of people carrying genes for harmful conditions. Present technology makes it possible to do this for a number of genetic diseases. Even when the specific gene responsible for the condition has not been isolated, a potential problem can be detected by studying many members of a family in which the disease has occurred over several generations. As part of this process, scientists cut chromosomes into segments using *restriction enzymes*, which slice DNA at specific sites. It has been found that the pattern of chromosome fragments in a family member carrying the faulty gene usually can be distinguished from the pattern in people who do not have the gene. The technique is not perfect, but it can be more than 90% accurate in determining whether an individual carries a specific gene.

The dilemmas that can arise from the ability to identify genetic defects are best illustrated in the case of Huntington's chorea. As previously mentioned, this disease causes progressive and untreatable degeneration of the nervous system starting in adult life. The ultimately fatal condition is caused by a dominant gene. (Huntington's victims include the legendary folksinger Woody Guthrie, 1912–67.)

It is now possible, however, to conduct a family analysis and tell people if they are carriers long before symptoms appear. However, even though detection of Huntington's chorea is possible, treatment is not. That means that individuals who have a parent with Huntington's chorea—and who therefore have a 50% risk of inheriting the gene for the condition—must decide whether they want to know if they too will face this slow, inevitable death. Many do not, saying they would rather live with uncertainty. Others do, believing that the knowledge will help them decide whether to marry and have children or to make the necessary preparations if the news is bad.

Many more Americans will probably face this sort of choice in the future. Genetic testing is expanding rapidly, and so is the number of genetic conditions that can be detected. Moreover, if, as predicted, the Human Genome Project enables doctors to identify thousands of gene mutations, the dilemma over how much a patient should know about his or her own inherited makeup is likely to intensify.

GENETIC TESTING AND
THE WORKPLACE

New insight into genetic disease will probably have financial repercussions in the future as well. Employers and insurance companies are starting to make decisions about hiring and issuing policies on the basis of individual genetic makeup. An example is *polycystic kidney disease*, an inherited condition caused by a dominant gene that leads to progressive kidney failure in adult life. Some insurance companies are requir-

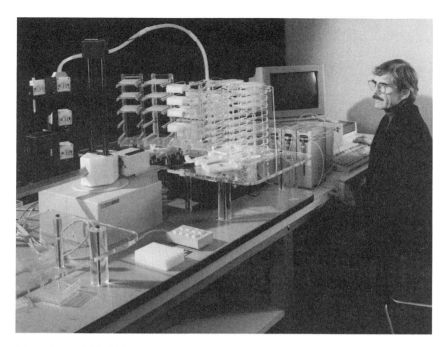

Mapping all 50,000 to 100,000 human genes will prove a daunting task; to help speed up the process, scientists are using this computer-controlled robot to help isolate fragments of human genetic material.

ing applicants born into families in which the disease occurs to be tested before a policy is issued. Similar restrictions on insurance coverage are being applied in a number of cases where genetic makeup influences health.

Ultimately, those limitations could affect virtually everyone. It has become clear that most chronic diseases of later life, such as heart disease and cancer, are under some sort of genetic influence. Researchers have identified genes that either increase the risk or provide protection against such conditions, and some companies are starting to test potential employees to weed out those whose genetic background might result in higher medical costs. The American Medical Association's Council on Scientific Affairs reported in December 1990 that "the potential for employers to abuse genetic testing and discriminate against individuals applying for employment is great."

Society does, however, have some time to prepare for the issues raised by genetic testing. Dr. Philip Reilly, director of the Shriver Center for Mental Retardation in Waltham, Massachusetts, and an expert on genetic testing, estimated in 1991 that mass testing of genetic makeup to predict the risk of heart disease and cancer would not be possible for 5 to 10 years. But in that time period, society must make decisions not only about genetic testing but also about prenatal screening and gene therapy, all of which will have a profound effect not only on the babies of tomorrow but also on the life and livelihood of many people.

Some ethicists have pointed to the specter of widespread use of prenatal screening and genetic testing to identify every possible abnormality in an unborn child. Some parents would feel compelled to end any pregnancy in which the fetus did not meet their standard of perfection, critics say. Even today, some couples have used prenatal detection for sex selection, first learning whether the unborn child is male or female and then deciding to continue the pregnancy only if the baby is the desired sex.

These issues at the frontiers of medicine and biology deserve widespread debate. Today's high school students will become parents in an era when the applications of biomedical technology are wider than ever before in history. The ethical and moral issues that accompany that technology cannot be left to scientists alone.

CHAPTER 9

HELP

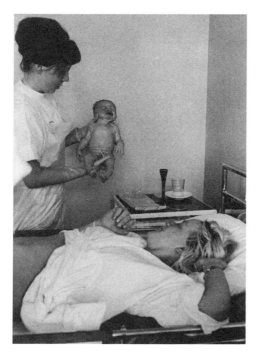

Millions of healthy infants are born in the United States each year, but for those suffering from defects, medical intervention can begin as early as birth.

M uch can be done to help children who are confronted with the risk of birth defects. Sometimes defects can be prevented, and in other cases their effects can be lessened by treatment. Often, better care can ease a lifetime burden.

EARLY INTERVENTION

One key is early intervention—quick identification of a problem, followed by the necessary steps to provide help. Depending on the problem, "early" can mean the first minutes or hours after birth, or it can mean during the first years of school. Sometimes many years of help are needed to counter the problems resulting from a birth defect.

Spina Bifida

For spina bifida, intervention must occur at the moment of birth. Because the spinal cord is exposed, it has been suggested that the battering that a baby takes during delivery can make the paralysis associated with this condition even worse. But a study reported in 1991 by physicians at the Swedish Hospital Medical Center in Seattle indicates that severe paralysis could be reduced if babies with spina bifida were delivered by cesarean section. Longer-term damage can be reduced by surgery to repair the hole in the spine immediately after birth.

Low Birthweight Babies

Low birthweight babies also require immediate intervention, in this case to prevent permanent lung damage. When babies are born prematurely, their lungs often are not ready to breathe because they lack a natural substance called *surfactant* that helps the lungs expand to receive air. The resulting condition, called *respiratory distress syndrome* or *hyaline membrane disease*, is the most common cause of death and disability in premature babies, affecting about 50,000 newborns in the United States each year and killing 5,000 of them. A new therapy, however, promises to reduce that toll significantly. The treatment uses an artificial surfactant that is sprayed into the newborn's lungs immediately after birth. In a typical study, reported in 1989, use of artificial surfactant reduced the incidence of permanent lung damage by 13%.

Fetal Surgery

Thanks to advancing technology, early intervention can also mean surgery to repair damage in a child before he or she is born, although the success of such procedures varies. For example, in February 1991, researchers from the University of California at San Francisco reported in the *Journal of the American Medical Association* on a series of 17 fetal operations performed over the previous decade to repair several different conditions. These included *diaphragmatic hernia*, a hole in the wall separating the abdomen and the chest; urinary tract blockage; a growth on the fetus's tailbone; and a growth in the unborn child's lung. In these operations, surgeons were able to literally open the womb and partially remove the fetus for surgery on the defective area. Unfortunately, some of the results were disappointing. Three of the operations ended in abortion when surgery failed and the fetus died.

Although eating healthy foods is important for every child, for youngsters suffering from conditions such as phenylketonuria and galactosemia, a special diet is essential to prevent mental retardation.

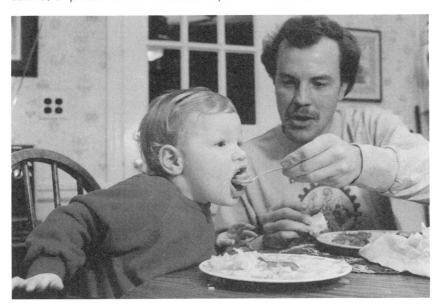

Another died 15 hours after the operation and a few died at birth. However, several of these operations did result in healthy children. It was also found that none of the mothers suffered serious injury and the surgery appeared to have no effect on their ability to have more children.

NUTRITION-RELATED INTERVENTION

Sometimes intervention against birth defects takes the form of a special diet. Such is the case for the condition known as *phenylketonuria*, or PKU, which leaves a child unable to metabolize an amino acid called *phenylalanine*, and for the defect called *galactosemia*, in which the body cannot use *galactose*, a sugar found in milk. A child with either condition who eats a normal diet will suffer progressive mental retardation.

A youngster with PKU, however, can be protected from the disease's effects through a low-protein diet, and a child with galactosemia can receive similar help via a diet that excludes milk sugar. Wilson's disease, a genetic condition that causes copper to accumulate in the liver, is treated by eliminating all foods with a high copper content from the diet, including chocolate, cherries, and beef. Otherwise this disorder can cause severe liver and brain damage. Sticking to these special diets requires great discipline but can prevent devastating problems. About a dozen genetic defects related to the body's metabolism, all of which are rare, can be detected by blood tests done in the first days after birth.

INTERVENTION AND EDUCATION

Early detection and treatment of one kind or another can help most children born with handicaps. A study in 1986 by the Colorado Department of Education showed that prompt assistance allowed a third of 1,300 children with disabilities to begin school without additional intervention. Another third of the children required only minimal help to attend school. But almost all the children whose handicaps were not identified early, and therefore did not receive quick attention, required full-time special education when they reached their school years.

THE APGAR SCORE

Deciding whether a child needs special intervention starts during pregnancy. Doctors look for the known risk factors—lack of prenatal care, use of drugs or alcohol by the mother, diabetes, or other trouble signs. The assessment continues at birth, when the obstetrician checks the newborn using the *Apgar score*, devised by an American physician, Virginia Apgar. The doctor scores five features at one minute and five minutes after birth: breathing effort, heart rate, color, muscle tone, and reflexes, with breathing and heart rate the most important. Each feature receives a numerical score. A score of 7 to 10 indicates a healthy baby, but 0 to 4 shows that emergency help is needed. Babies who score from 5 to 7 usually do not require major help.

Research indicates that in many cases early intervention reduces the amount of special help handicapped children need when they start school.

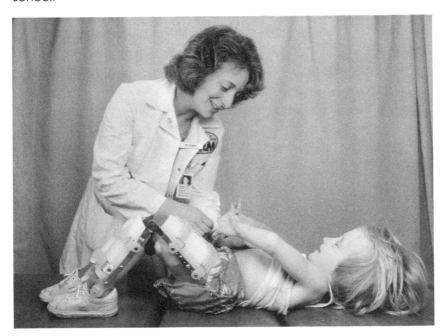

MARY BOSS

In many ways, 17-year-old Mary Boss is like other adolescents. The oldest of four children, she has a penchant for reading *Teen* magazine, is a member of the high school chorus, and knows her way around a computer keyboard, touch-typing about 25 to 30 words per minute. But in other respects Mary is not typical: The Greenwood Lake, New York, teenager has Down's syndrome.

Despite her accomplishments, when Mary was born in 1974, her parents, Bill and Barbara, had little way of knowing the extent of their daughter's potential. There simply was not much helpful information on the abilities of children with Down's syndrome. At the hospital where Mary was born, says Barbara, the Bosses received only one piece of advice: "She's your daughter. Take her home and love her."

A few months after their daughter's birth, the Bosses began to see a genetic counselor. They were also given the name of a support group consisting of parents of children with Down's syndrome, but Barbara was uneasy about joining. "I couldn't even deal with [Mary's condition] myself," she says, "much less talk to someone else about it."

When Barbara finally contacted the support group, however, she found the first ray of hope in her family's difficult situation. Speaking to a mother whose three-year-old child was toilet trained and talking, Barbara became encouraged by the possibilities for Mary's development.

The Bosses sought out other programs designed to give Mary the special help she needed, although at the time not many such early intervention plans were available. With the aid of these programs, the Bosses encouraged Mary's mental and physical development. Early intervention included making certain that there were colorful, stimulating toys in Mary's crib. It was also important to provide her with strength-building exercises, because infants with Down's syndrome tend to lack proper muscle tone. As a baby, Mary had trouble supporting her head, so her parents helped to strengthen her neck muscles by hanging mobiles above her, objects to catch her attention and to encourage her to look up. The Bosses also encouraged Mary to perform crawling motions, moving her arms and legs in an effort to develop these muscles as well.

Even dressing their daughter became a learning activity. "You had to make sure the child was involved with what you were doing," says Barbara. This meant teaching the baby to participate in the dressing procedure, to "get an exchange rather than having this passive child just laying there."

"What we tried to do was to speak to her as much as possible and encourage everyone else in our family and in our extended family to also speak to her rather than speak around her," says Bill. This not only boosted Mary's language skills but apparently helped others come to terms with her condition.

Today, Mary attends high school, where, according to her father, she is a conscientious and highly organized student. Like many other children with Down's syndrome, she has been *mainstreamed*, which in her case means that she is combining typical classes in subjects such as computer education and physical fitness with special courses in some of the stricter academic topics, including English, math, and science. At home her responsibilities include chores such as doing laundry and caring for the family dog.

As society's doors open for people with handicaps, adults with Down's syndrome are carving their niche in the workplace as well. According to the National Down Syndrome Society, people with Down's syndrome are finding employment everywhere, from offices to nursing homes to restaurants.

As children with Down's syndrome are mainstreamed, it has become apparent that bringing up a teenager with the condition is often much like raising other adolescents. For example, like most 17 year olds, Mary dreams of driving a car. "My own red Corvette with a sunroof," she says.

Yet Mary's handicap makes such situations a little bit different, says her mother. "Like when it comes to other kids, when they get to be 16, generally that means you go out and get your driver's license. . . . And Mary isn't quite ready for that."

Mary's choices for the future are as varied as any of her peers'. She is thinking of becoming a beautician or perhaps a photographer. "I want to do almost everything," she says. But people with Down's syndrome continue to face an important question, says her father, because they must wonder, "whether or not doors might be opened or closed before [they're] even given a chance to prove [themselves]."

NEWBORN INTENSIVE CARE

A study published in 1989 by the American Hospital Association indicated that at least 668 hospitals had neonatal intensive care units (ICUs), facilities specially designed for newborns who need life-saving help. Babies with low Apgar scores, those with low birthweight, and those with infections or other problems are placed in these units for treatment. If the baby has trouble breathing, for example, it will be given oxygen. Those with low blood sugar are given glucose. *Jaundice*, a condition caused by low liver function, is treated by bathing the baby in light. (Jaundice is caused by the accumulation of *bilirubin*, a substance that normally is metabolized by the liver. Light therapy is believed to stimulate breakdown of the chemical.) Anemia in a newborn is treated with iron supplements or, in severe cases, blood transfusions. A newborn intensive care unit is equipped with special cribs called *isolettes*, where a variety of different treatments can be administered. A stay in one of these ICUs is expensive, however, costing as much as $30,000 for an infant who is well below normal birthweight.

HIDDEN HANDICAPS

Although some handicaps are apparent at birth, others do not become obvious until later in a child's life. Therefore, early screening to detect hidden problems is recommended for all young children. One widely used method is the *Denver Developmental Screening Test*, which can be administered in 15 to 20 minutes. The child is evaluated on the basis of simple abilities, such as using a spoon, helping in the house, putting one block on top of another, naming pictures, kicking a ball, and so on. The test has been found to identify up to 85% of children with developmental problems. Once a problem is identified, the child should be referred to a specialized center for individual care.

Unfortunately, many doctors do not use such screening tests. A 1986 study found that only 39% of pediatricians and 29% of family doctors did routine evaluations to determine whether children were developing normally. As a result, it appears that many children who need help do not receive it early enough for maximum effectiveness.

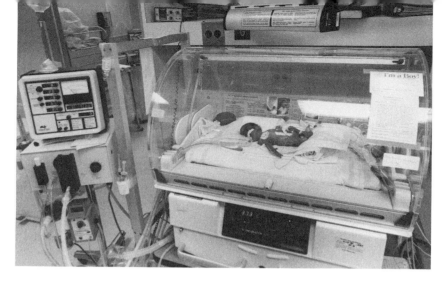

Newborn intensive care units can be found in hundreds of hospitals across the United States. These facilities can treat premature and low-birthweight infants for a variety of problems, including breathing difficulties, low blood sugar, and jaundice.

LIFESAVING ADVANCES

Some conditions inevitably require lifetime attention but do yield to new advances. For example, the life span of children born with cystic fibrosis once was only a few years, and survival beyond adolescence was rare. Today, many cystic fibrosis patients live for decades. The disease causes a deficiency in pancreatic enzymes that are essential for digestion and also an accumulation of an especially thick mucus in the throat, which leaves patients extremely vulnerable to infection.

Now, however, enzyme tablets can help digestion. The threat of infection is reduced by having cystic fibrosis patients do a methodical, thorough clearing of the mucus every day, and antibiotics are given at the earliest sign of infection. The isolation of the gene for cystic fibrosis in 1989 has allowed scientists to learn more about the molecular basis of the disease, opening the way for new forms of treatment.

The quality and length of life have also improved for individuals with Down's syndrome. At the beginning of the century, most children with Down's syndrome died before the age of 10, usually from infections. Antibiotics doubled the age of survival, and better treatment of all aspects of the condition now allows many individuals with Down's syndrome to live into their sixties and seventies.

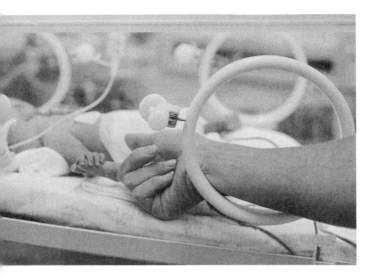

Despite the many hurdles faced by handicapped children, love, care, and advancing medical technology offer hope in the war against birth defects.

Longer survival, however, might not count for much without an accompanying change of attitude toward people with Down's syndrome. It was once commonly thought that a youngster with Down's syndrome had no useful role in society and had to be placed in an institution for care. Now it has become apparent that systematic schooling and attentive home care can allow these children to reach their true potential.

Indeed, this type of acceptance plays an essential part in the war against birth defects. Medical diagnosis and treatment, no matter how advanced, may never prevent every reproductive problem. Therefore it is important for people to understand that a physically imperfect individual can lead a productive life. If employers, insurers, and educators resolve to help meet the needs of the handicapped and those whose genetic makeup places them at risk for disease, society will have come a long way in reducing the fear and trauma associated with birth defects.

APPENDIX:
FOR MORE INFORMATION

The following is a list of organizations that can provide further information about birth defects and related topics.

GENERAL INFORMATION

Alliance of Genetic Support Groups
1001 22nd Street NW
Suite 800
Washington, DC 20037
(202) 331-0942 (in Washington, DC)
(800) 336-GENE (outside Washington, DC)

American Society of Human Genetics
9650 Rockville Pike
Bethesda, MD 20814
(301) 571-1825

Association of Birth Defect Children
5400 Diplomat Circle
Suite 270
Orlando, FL 32810
(407) 629-1466

Canadian Foundation for the Study of Infant Deaths
586 Eglinton Avenue East
Suite 308
Toronto, Ontario M4P 1P2
Canada
(416) 488-3260

International Council of Guilds for Infant Survival
9178 Nadine River Circle
Fountain Valley, CA 92708
(714) 968-7623 (in California)
(800) 247-4370 (outside California)

March of Dimes Birth Defects Foundation
1275 Mamaroneck Avenue
White Plains, NY 10605
(914) 428-7100

National Center for Clinical Infant Programs
2000 14th Street N
Suite 380
Arlington, VA 22201
(703) 528-4300

National Commission to Prevent Infant Mortality
Switzer Building
Room 2014
330 C Street SW
Washington, DC 20201
(202) 472-1364

National Network to Prevent Birth
  Defects
Box 15309
Southeast Station
Washington, DC 20003
(202) 543-5450

National Organization for Rare
  Disorders, Inc.
P.O. Box 8923
New Fairfield, CT 06812
(203) 746-6518 (in Connecticut)
(800) 999-6673 (outside Connecticut)

CANCER

American Cancer Society
1599 Clifton Road NE
Atlanta, GA 30329
(800) 227-2345

Canadian Cancer Society
10 Alcorn Avenue
Toronto, Ontario M4V 3B1
Canada
(416) 961-7223

Leukemia Society of America, Inc.
733 Third Avenue
New York, NY 10017
(212) 573-8484

National Cancer Care Foundation
1180 Avenue of the Americas
New York, NY 10036
(212) 221-3300

CEREBRAL PALSY

United Cerebral Palsy Associations,
  Inc./UCP Research and Educational
  Foundation
7 Penn Plaza
Suite 804
New York, NY 10001

(212) 268-6655 (in New York)
(800) USA-1UCP (outside New York)

CLEFT PALATE

American Cleft Palate Association/The
  Cleft Palate Foundation
1218 Grandview Avenue
Pittsburgh, PA 15211
(412) 481-1376 (in Pennsylvania)
(800) 24-CLEFT (outside Pennsylvania)

CRI-DU-CHAT SYNDROME

5p- Society
11609 Oakmont
Overland Park, KS 66201
(913) 469-8900

DIABETES

American Diabetes Assocation, Inc.
1660 Duke Street
Alexandria, VA 22314
(800) 232-3472

Juvenile Diabetes Foundation
  International
432 Park Avenue South
16th Floor
New York, NY 10010
(212) 889-7575
(212) JDF-CURE

DOMINANT GENE DEFECTS

Hereditary Disease Foundation
1427 Seventh Street
Suite 2
Santa Monica, CA 90401
(213) 458-4183

Huntington's Disease Society of
  America, Inc.
140 West Twenty-second Street
New York, NY 10011-2420

(212) 242-1968 (in New York)
(800) 345-HDSA (outside New York)

National Marfan Foundation
382 Main Street
Port Washington, NY 11050
(516) 883-8712

DOWN'S SYNDROME

Association for Children with Down
    Syndrome, Inc.
2616 Martin Avenue
Bellmore, NY 11710
(516) 221-4700

National Down Syndrome Congress
1800 Dempster Street
Park Ridge, IL 60068-1146
(708) 823-7550 (in Illinois)
(800) 232-NDSC (outside Illinois)

National Down Syndrome Society
666 Broadway
New York, NY 10012
(212) 460-9330 (in New York)
(800) 221-4602 (outside New York)

EPILEPSY

Epilepsy Foundation of America
4351 Garden City Drive
Landover, MD 20785
(301) 459-3700

HEMOPHILIA

National Hemophilia Foundation
The Soho Building
110 Greene Street
Room 303
New York, NY 10012
(212) 219-8180

LEARNING DISABILITIES

Learning Disabilities Association of
    America
4156 Library Road
Pittsburgh, PA 15234
(412) 341-1515

Orton Dyslexia Society
Chester Building
Suite 382
8600 LaSalle Road
Baltimore, MD 21204-6020
(301) 296-0232 (in Maryland)
(800) ABCD-123 (outside Maryland)

MENTAL RETARDATION

Association for Retarded Citizens of the
    United States
P.O. Box 1047
Arlington, TX 76004
(817) 261-6003

MONOSOMY

Support Group for Monosomy 9p
43304 Kipton Nickel Plate Road
La Grange, OH 44050
(216) 775-4255

MUSCULAR DYSTROPHY

Muscular Dystrophy Assocation
3561 East Sunrise Drive
Tucson, AZ 85718
(602) 529-2000 (in Arizona)
(800) 223-6666 (outside Arizona)

NEUROFIBROMATOSIS

National Neurofibromatosis Founda-
    tion, Inc.
141 Fifth Avenue
Suite 7-S

New York, NY 10010
(212) 460-8980 (in New York)
(800) 323-7938 (outside New York)

RECESSIVE GENE DEFECTS

Cystic Fibrosis Foundation
6931 Arlington Road
Bethesda, MD 20814
(301) 951-4422 (in Maryland)
(800) FIGHT CF (outside Maryland)

National Tay-Sachs and Allied Diseases
  Association, Inc.
2001 Beacon Street
Suite 304
Brookline, MA 02146
(617) 227-4463

SICKLE-CELL ANEMIA

National Association for Sickle Cell
  Disease, Inc.
3345 Wilshire Boulevard
Suite 1106
Los Angeles, CA 90010-1880

(213) 736-5455 (in California)
(800) 421-8453 (outside California)

SPINA BIFIDA

Spina Bifida Association of America
1700 Rockville Pike
Suite 250
Rockville, MD 20852
(301) 770-7222 (in Maryland)
(800) 621-3141 (outside Maryland)

WILSON'S DISEASE

National Foundation for Study of
  Wilson's Disease
5447 Palisade Avenue
Bronx, NY 10471
(212) 430-2091

Wilson's Disease Association
P.O. Box 75324
Washington, DC 20013
(703) 636-3003
(703) 636-3014

FURTHER READING

GENERAL INFORMATION

Bergsma, Daniel, and Brian R. Lowry, eds. *Natural History of Specific Birth Defects*. New York: Liss, 1977.

Evers-Kiebooms, Gerry, et al., eds. *Genetic Risk, Risk Perception, and Decision Making*. New York: Liss, 1987.

Feingold, Murray, and Hermione Pashayan. *Genetics and Birth Defects in Clinical Practice*. Boston: Little, Brown, 1983.

Goodman, Richard M., and Robert J. Gorlin. *The Malformed Infant and Child: An Illustrated Guide*. New York: Oxford University Press, 1983.

Huffstadt, A. J. *Congenital Malformations*. New York: Elsevier, 1981.

Jones, Kenneth L. *Smith's Recognizable Patterns of Human Malformation*. 4th ed. Philadelphia: Saunders, 1988.

Kelly, Sally, et al., eds. *Birth Defects: Risks and Consequences*. San Diego: Academic Press, 1976.

Kolb Meyers, V., ed. *Teratogens: Chemicals Which Cause Birth Defects*. New York: Elsevier, 1988.

Nurnberger, John I., ed. *Biological and Environmental Determinants of Early Development*. New York: Raven Press, 1973.

Persaud, T. V. *Genetic Disorders, Syndromology, and Prenatal Diagnosis.* New York: Liss, 1982.

Simmons, Jackie A. *Minor Birth Defects.* Lorain, OH: Dayton Laboratories, 1978.

Sparks, Shirley N. *Birth Defects and Speech-Language Disorders.* Boston: College-Hill, 1984.

Sucheston, Martha E., and M. Samuel Cannon. *Congenital Malformations: Case Studies in Developmental Anatomy.* Philadelphia: Davis, 1973.

Taffel, Selma. *Congenital Abnormalities and Birth Injuries Among Live Birth.* Edited by Arlett Brown. Hyattsville, MD: National Center For Health Statistics, 1978.

CEREBRAL PALSY

Galjaard, H., et al., eds. *Early Detection and Management of Cerebral Palsy.* Norwell, MA: Kluwer Academic, 1987.

Hardy, James C. *Cerebral Palsy.* Englewood Cliffs, NJ: Prentice-Hall, 1983.

McDonald, Eugene T., ed. *Treating Cerebral Palsy.* Austin: Pro-Ed, 1987.

Schleichkorn, Jay. *Coping with Cerebral Palsy: Answers to Questions Parents Often Ask.* Austin: Pro-Ed, 1983.

CLEFT PALATE

Edwards, et al. *Advances in the Management of Cleft Palate.* New York: Churchill, 1981.

Starr, Philip, et al. *Cleft Lip and or Palate: Behavioral Effects from Infancy to Adulthood.* Springfield, IL: Thomas, 1983.

Wynn, Sidney K., and Alfred L. Miller, eds. *A Practical Guide to Cleft Lip and Palate Birth Defects: Helpful Practical Information and Answers for Parents, Physicians, Nurses and Other Professionals.* Springfield, IL: Thomas, 1984.

DIABETES

Laron, Z., ed. *Prognosis of Diabetes in Children.* New York: Karger, 1988.

Lauffer, Ira J., and Herbert Kadison. *Diabetes Explained: A Layman's Guide.* New York: Dutton, 1976.

Mimura, G., ed. *Childhood and Juvenile Diabetes Mellitus.* New York: Elsevier, 1986.

DOWN'S SYNDROME

Cunningham, Cliff. *Down's Syndrome: An Introduction for Parents.* Cambridge, MA: Brookline Books, 1982.

Dmitriev, Val, and Pat Oelwein, eds. *Advances in Down Syndrome.* Seattle: Special Child Publications, 1988.

Pueschel, Siegfried. *An Overview of Down Syndrome.* Arlington, TX: Association for Retarded Citizens of the United States, 1986.

HEMOPHILIA

Forbes, C. D. *Unresolved Problems in Haemophilia.* Norwell, MA: Kluwer Academic, 1981.

Jones, Peter. *Living with Hemophilia.* 3rd ed. Norwell, MA: Kluwer Academic, N. d.

LEARNING DISABILITIES

Bakker, D., et al., eds. *Developmental Dyslexia and Learning Disorders.* New York: Karger, 1987.

Bergsma, Daniel, ed. *X-Linked Mental Retardation and Verbal Disability.* White Plains, NY: March of Dimes, N. d.

Bryan, Tanis H., and James H. Bryan. *Understanding Learning Disabilities.* Mountain View, CA: Mayfield, 1986.

MUSCULAR DYSTROPHY

Douglas, Ruben H., and Nancy R. Macciomei, eds. *Muscular Dystrophy: Readings.* White Plains, NY: Longman, 1986.

Ebashi, Setsuro, ed. *Muscular Dystrophy.* New York: Columbia University Press, 1983.

SICKLE-CELL ANEMIA

Edelstein, Stuart J. *The Sickled Cell.* Cambridge: Harvard University Press, 1986.

Serjeant, Graham R. *Sickle Cell Disease.* New York: Oxford University Press, 1986.

SPINA BIFIDA

Dobing, John, ed. *Prevention of Spina Bifida and Other Neural Tube Defects.* San Diego: Academic Press, 1983.

McLaurin, Robert L., et al., eds. *Spina Bifida: A Multidisciplinary Approach.* New York: Praeger, 1986.

GLOSSARY

Agent Orange an herbicide, used as a defoliant during the Vietnam War, that may be linked to birth defects found in children of veterans exposed to the chemical

amniocentesis the insertion of a needle through the abdominal wall and into the uterus to remove amniotic fluid; the fetal cells in the liquid are then examined to determine the sex of the fetus and to detect any abnormalities

amniotic fluid the liquid found in the womb that protects the fetus from injury

anencephaly the congenital absence of all or a major part of the brain

anticoagulants a group of drugs administered to reduce blood clotting; have been found capable of damaging a fetus's bones and cartilage and can result in fetal blindness, mental retardation, and stillbirth

anticonvulsants a group of drugs used to relieve epilepsy that have been associated with an increased risk of birth defects

Apgar score a system used to record an infant's physical condition (respiration, heart rate, color, muscle tone, and reflexes) one minute and five minutes after birth

cerebral palsy a nervous system disorder resulting from damage that occurs before or during birth; leaves the child partially paralyzed and suffering from poor muscle coordination

cesarean section the surgical removal of the fetus through the abdomen

chorionic villi sampling the removal of villi (tiny fingerlike projections found in the uterus) during the early stages of pregnancy to test for possible birth defects

chromosomes rodlike structures of DNA and protein found in the nuclei of cells; each normal human cell contains 23 pairs of chromosomes

cleft palate birth defect characterized by an opening in the palate (roof of the mouth) that forms a passageway between the nasal cavity and the mouth

congenital present at birth

cystic fibrosis an inherited disease that affects the pancreas, respiratory system, and sweat glands; characterized by chronic respiratory infections and problems absorbing food

Denver Developmental Screening Test a test administered to young children that uses simple mental and physical tests to determine whether a youngster's development has been delayed

DES diethylstilbestrol; a sex hormone, prescribed during the 1960s to prevent miscarriage, that was later found to increase risk of genital cancer to female children exposed to DES in the womb

diploid cells that contain two sets of chomosomes

DNA deoxyribonucleic acid; genetic material that contains chemical instructions for determining an organism's inherited characteristics

dominant a characteristic that appears in an offspring even though the child received that trait from the genes of only one parent

Down's syndrome trisomy 21; usually caused by the presence of an extra chromosome 21; characterized by a sloping forehead, slanting eyes, flat nose, dwarfed physique, and moderate to severe mental retardation

dyslexia a condition that, independent of intelligence and vision, affects a person's ability to read

fragile-X syndrome the most common inherited cause of mental retardation; results from a weakness in an abnormal X chromosome that causes it to break

genes complex units of chemical material contained within the chromosomes; variations in the patterns formed by the components of genes are responsible for inherited traits

genetic counseling the application of genetics to educate individuals about the probability of producing children with hereditary abnormalities; a physician or counselor studies the genetic family history of both the mother and father to arrive at a conclusion

haploid sex cells; cells that contain a single set of chromosomes

hemophilia a sex-linked hereditary disease, found almost exclusively in males, in which the blood does not clot properly, causing even minor injuries to result in severe hemorrhaging (uncontrollable bleeding)

incomplete penetrance a genetic phenomenon that occurs when an individual inherits the mutated genes of a dominant condition but does not develop all symptoms of the disease

Klinefelter's syndrome a condition, suffered only by males born with an extra X chromosome, that causes sterility and mental retardation and may result in a feminine appearance

Marfan syndrome a dominant gene defect characterized by a tall lean body, long fingers and toes, stooped shoulders, flat feet, and abnormal joint flexibility; often, the aorta will become dilated and weaken, allowing an aneurysm to develop

MSAFP maternal serum alpha-fetoprotein screening test; a prenatal blood test performed in the 16th to 18th week of pregnancy in which the mother's blood is analyzed for alpha-fetoprotein (AFP); excessive or low levels of AFP indicate various types of birth defects, including Down's syndrome, and may indicate that a child will be stillborn

meiosis the process through which the body's sex cells divide to create gametes (sperm or ova); successive divisions of the nucleus produce human cells containing 23 chromosomes—half the number of chromosomes present in other cells

meiotic nondisjunction an error occurring during meiosis in which a pair of chromosomes fails to separate

miscarriage abortion of the fetus by the mother's body

mitosis the process by which cells (excluding the sex cells) pass on their genetic material during cell division; the new cells formed contain as many chromosomes as did the parent cells

mitotic nondisjunction an error occurring during mitosis in which certain cells divide improperly resulting in some cells lacking one chromosome and some having an extra chromosome

monosomy a lethal condition characterized by the absence of a single chromosome

muscular dystrophy a disease causing progressive weakening and atrophy of the muscles

placenta the organ through which the fetus receives its food; connects the fetus to the uterus

placental abruption premature detachment of the placenta from the wall of the womb; can be caused by smoking during pregnancy

prenatal before birth

recessive a characteristic that will appear in an offspring only if the child received the genes of that trait from both parents

sickle-cell anemia an inherited blood disease in which some red blood cells sickle, or form into crescent shapes; can be fatal

SIDS sudden infant death syndrome; commonly known as crib death; the unexplained death of an apparently healthy baby, usually occurring between the second week and first year of life

spina bifida a birth defect in which the walls of the spinal canal do not close completely, leaving the spinal cord partially exposed and at risk of injury during delivery

stillbirth the birth of a dead fetus

syndrome a group of symptoms or defects occurring together

Tay-Sachs disease a fatal inherited condition characterized by mental and physical retardation; the outcome of a lack of the enzyme hexosamidase A, which aids in the breakdown of fat

thalidomide a sedative and sleeping pill the use of which was discontinued when it was discovered that intake of the drug during pregnancy resulted in malformation of the arms and legs in developing fetuses

trisomy a condition in which 1 sex cell contains 24 chromosomes; if fertilization occurs with this cell, an abnormal embryo will be produced

Turner's syndrome the absence of an X chromosome in females; can result in short stature, sterility, and various learning disorders

ultrasound a prenatal diagnostic test that uses high-frequency sound waves to generate images of a fetus

INDEX

PICTURE CREDITS

The Bettmann Archive: pp. 14, 81, 85; Food and Drug Administration: p. 67; Courtesy of George Washington Medical Center: p. 41 (left and right); cover: ICON Communications/FPG; Courtesy of March of Dimes: pp. 27, 28, 30; Courtesy of March of Dimes, Birth Defects Foundation: pp. 16, 18, 24, 32, 47, 54, 93, 94; National Cancer Institute, National Institutes of Health: p. 78 (left: photo by Brooks Studio; right: photo by Bill Branson); National Institute of Child Health and Human Development, National Institutes of Health: pp. 13, 19, 33, 45, 61, 71, 72, 87, 89; National Institutes of Health: pp. 56, 80; National Library of Medicine: p. 25; Reuters/Bettmann Archive: p. 51; Courtesy of Stanford University Medical Center: p. 69; Gary Tong: pp. 23, 35, 36, 37, 38, 39, 43; University of California, Lawrence Berkeley Lab: pp. 77, 83; UPI/Bettmann Archive: pp. 21, 48, 53, 58, 60, 63, 65, 75; U.S. Department of Agriculture: p. 49

Edward Edelson is former science editor of the *New York Daily News* and past president of the National Association of Science Writers. His books include *The ABC's of Prescription Narcotics* and the textbook *Chemical Principles*. He has won awards for his writing from such groups as the American Heart Association, the American Cancer Society, the American Academy of Pediatrics, and the American Psychological Society.

Dale C. Garell, M.D., is medical director of California Children Services, Department of Health Services, County of Los Angeles. He is also associate dean for curriculum at the University of Southern California School of Medicine and clinical professor in the Department of Pediatrics & Family Medicine at the University of Southern California School of Medicine. From 1963 to 1974, he was medical director of the Division of Adolescent Medicine at Children's Hospital in Los Angeles. Dr. Garell has served as president of the Society for Adolescent Medicine, chairman of the youth committee of the American Academy of Pediatrics, and as a forum member of the White House Conference on Children (1970) and White House Conference on Youth (1971). He has also been a member of the editorial board of the *American Journal of Diseases of Children*.

C. Everett Koop, M.D., Sc.D., is former Surgeon General, deputy assistant secretary for health, and director of the Office of International Health of the U.S. Public Health Service. A pediatric surgeon with an international reputation, he was previously surgeon-in-chief of Children's Hospital of Philadelphia and professor of pediatric surgery and pediatrics at the University of Pennsylvania. Dr. Koop is the author of more than 175 articles and books on the practice of medicine. He has served as surgery editor of the *Journal of Clinical Pediatrics* and editor-in-chief of the *Journal of Pediatric Surgery*. Dr. Koop has received nine honorary degrees and numerous other awards, including the Denis Brown Gold Medal of the British Association of Paediatric Surgeons, the William E. Ladd Gold Medal of the American Academy of Pediatrics, and the Copernicus Medal of the Surgical Society of Poland. He is a chevalier of the French Legion of Honor and a member of the Royal College of Surgeons, London.